For all the women out there who are going through the miracle of pregnancy at this moment.

Cover design by J. Meier

First Printing: October 2010

ISBN- 978-1-4461-2601-1

Alternative Therapies in Pregnancy

By Jennifer Meier

Foreword

I have been pondering on whether to write this book for over two years now, at first I wanted to write it while I was pregnant, as a sort of Diary, but in the end I couldn't because of some pregnancy symptoms that made my last pregnancy a wee bit of a burden. Don't get me wrong, it was a wonderful experience, but during the second month, my mother in law died. It wasn't so much the sadness and grief that got to me, but more the burden of having to clean out her rented apartment. We filled seven skips and twenty three large rubbish bags, and that was after opening the apartment to scavengers! Or at least telling people to take what they wanted. I never would have thought somebody could fit so much junk into one small space, but she did and a lot of it was heavy. So after hauling so many books and junk, I got a kidney that threatened to fail on me, and a small tear in my womb. SO after that I pretty much didn't do anything! But I got to really get in touch with myself, and to really enjoy my other two children before the demands of a new baby would start diverting my attention.

This book was conceived while I searched for books during each of my three pregnancies. I found a lot of books but none of them covered all the topics I wanted. So I had several books on oils, several on homeopathy and several more telling me how my baby was developing. There are many books on separate topics, so I decided to try combine the different alternative therapies available to a pregnant women. I don't like taking pills at all, so during my pregnancy it was a definite no.

Table of Contents

Nine Months

Maybe you've just found out that you're expecting, or maybe you're planning on getting pregnant, either way, I think it is important to understand what is happening to your body during this time. It is one of the most beautiful experiences woman will ever encounter, and yet one of the most trying. Since the dawn of time people have tried to understand the miracles of birth and death, and although we have learned during the past century or so, physically what happens, the spiritual side still remains a mystery.

As a mother of three, I went through my three pregnancies searching for various books on various subjects, and never seemed to be able to find "the right" book on pregnancy. So During my last pregnancy I took notes and recorded a lot of my research. I hope you, the reader, will find this information as useful as I have.

I've often pondered over how a baby comes to be, and still do, but I guess I will never fully understand the powers at work as a new human is being made. We can only guess at most of the questions concerning how the baby lives through the nine months, and I have often wondered when exactly the baby becomes fully aware, in saying this, I believe that when conception takes place, that the soul starts preparing for the decent to our world again, but that the consciousness does not become one with the baby at once, it must first align itself with the baby, slowdown it's vibration, and very slowly then merge with the body. I personally think it could be sometime around three months when the morning sickness normally starts to subside, but others argue that it would be at the actual birth.

I find it is important to talk to your baby during this time, in meditation or just by having a conversation with him or her, it not only helps the baby but can also help the mother by reducing stress and making her aware that she is never alone, and babies like to hear the voice of mommy, it's comforting for them. Meditation is important, especially during pregnancy as it will reduce stress, make you more aware of your body and keep you sane during all the mood swings, it will also help reduce fatigue, as you are completely relaxed during meditation, this gives your body quality time to adjust to the changing levels of work being done, saying this I should also tell you that a pregnant body during the first three months of pregnancy, works harder than a non-pregnant body climbing a mountain! Not that I ever climbed a mountain. Amazing, but true, so you see it's important to give your body a chance to rest completely.

The nine months of pregnancy are a most wonderful time to be enjoyed as much as possible, a time to share something so special with your partner that will bring you closer together. As a couple you will share in a miracle!

The First Month

About 5 to 7 days after a sperm fertilizes an egg, the egg attaches to the lining of the uterus, up to this time, the fertilized egg was just floating around!. This process is called implantation. The fertilized egg then begins to grow at a phenomenal rate in the uterus, doubling in size every day. At this stage of development the baby is called an embryo, it does not look very much like a human at the moment, but for every expecting mother, her embryo is still the cutest thing in the whole world!.

Shortly after implantation the placenta and umbilical cord begin to form. These are probably the two most important life giving things for your babies nine month stay in your womb. The placenta and umbilical cord provide nourishment and oxygen for your baby and carry away the baby's wastes, it is also the connection to you.

Your baby is enclosed in a sac of fluid, called the amniotic sac, to protect the baby from bumps and pressure, it bobs around in this sac, safe and sound away from the dangerous outside world.

In just another week the baby has a spinal cord. A few days later, five to eight bones of the spinal column (vertebrae) are in place. Nerve development is beginning. And by the end of your first 6 weeks of pregnancy, your baby has a head and trunk.

The embryo becomes three layers around the 5th week. The outer layer consists of the brain, nerves, and skin. The middle layer becomes the bones, muscles, blood vessels, heart, and sex organs. The inner layer holds the stomach, liver, intestines, lungs, and urinary tract. The eyes and other features begin to form, as do tiny buds that will be the arms and legs. The heart also forms, and it begins to beat on the 25th day after conception (5 to 6 weeks after the last menstrual period).

However, it is impossible to hear the heart beating at this time. This is something I once said to try and convince my sister not to abort her baby, I must say I'm extremely against abortion, and although my husband once said it would be better than bringing an unloved child to this world, I'm completely against it. Every child is loved by someone, I firmly believe that. However, I know many couples who cannot have children and would give anything to be given the chance to adopt an "unwanted" baby, even if it was born through rape. I also believe there is always a reason behind the conception of such a child, and I just can't bring myself to believe punishing the child (or embryo) is fair, as I see the beating of the heart as a sign of life, and to abort is to kill life sacred to the whatever god you believe in.

Anyway, as my sister wanted to abort her baby, I was disgusted, I don't believe in butting into other peoples affairs, but this was my nephew, I knew it would be a boy, I could feel it deep down inside me, and for me he was already alive. I managed to convince my sister, who now several years later, can't believe she ever thought of such a thing! My nephew is such a little darling, It was the best telling off she ever had, and she'll tell you that herself.

By the end of 6 weeks, your baby is about 1/2 inch long and weighs a fraction of an ounce. This is about the size of a kidney bean, yes so tiny.

What is Happening With You

At your first prenatal care appointment, or at the doctor's office to find out why you're not feeling so good! , your doctor will examine you to confirm your pregnancy and assess your health status, record your complete medical history, and give you some routine tests. That is after your doctor and the rest of the clinic staff have congratulated you on your tiny bump to be!

You may be given some of the following common prenatal tests:

- a pregnancy test; obviously
- a blood test to determine your blood type and to check for anaemia;
- urine analysis to screen for sugar, protein, white blood cells, blood, and bacteria;
- blood screens to determine immunity to diseases such as rubella;
- tests to disclose the presence of sexually transmitted infections and some other diseases;

- genetic tests for sickle-cell anaemia or Tay-Sachs disease;
- a Pap smear for the detection of cervical cancer; and/or
- a gestational diabetic screening test.

The tests you receive will depend on your personal and family medical history-you may not receive all of these tests. And you may choose not to have some of them. I personally just had to pee in a plastic cup and give one tube of blood.

And now to the "symptoms"...

During your first month of pregnancy, you may experience fatigue and sleepiness, falling asleep on your coffee break at work falls into this category! Frequent urination, nausea, vomiting, heartburn, indigestion, bloating, food aversions or cravings, and/or breast changes. In other words, you'll be tired and queezy. These pregnancy symptoms vary from woman to woman. You may experience all of them, just a few, or none of them.

Emotionally, you may feel irritable, have mood swings, may act irrationally, and be quick to cry. These emotions are similar to those experienced by women who have premenstrual syndrome. It is also common to have a variety of feelings about being pregnant, including misgivings, fear, joy, and elation. I think these changes get more pronounced with each pregnancy, my first was barely noticeable, but my third was difficult, I often cried for no reason, well actually, I did have reasons, they were just unreasonable! I once cried because they didn't have the bread I wanted at the bakery! And I often got the urge to hit people for little or no reason, which is totally unlike me, really! It's very strange sensation to not have complete control over your own body, but it gets better!

What is Happening With Your Partner

Your partner will also likely feel many different emotions about your pregnancy. It is normal for one or both of you to feel scared, upset, joyous, or a combination of all of these emotions. It is important to talk with each other about how you are feeling

Bach Flowers

I've decided to give this in the first chapter as a lot of the emotional changes start very early, you may become irritable before pregnancy is even confirmed, and as I always have a bottle of rescue remedy in my handbag for emergencies, I think Bach flowers are not just for this special time, but also for all the time.

Obviously, pregnancy is an ideal time to take the flower remedies, because it can be a time of great emotional upheaval, and sharp swings in mood. There is often a lot of fear and apprehension concerning the birth, for me it was more the fear I would end up giving birth in a hospital, which I wanted to avoid, and a need to deal with issues from the past, and prepare for the new transition.

I have found these remedies to be particularly helpful in pregnancy: Larch for confidence, Oak for inner strength, Aspen and Mimulus for fear and anxiety, Honeysuckle for letting go of the past, and Walnut for making the transition to motherhood, rescue remedy also helped me every time I had to do a blood test, as I have a fear of needles. I always took four drops just before going in to the nurse.

Dowsing for Child birth

It is also very helpful to dowse or Pendle a remedy for the labour and birth. It is impossible to predict what a labour will be like. Trust your instincts and the remedy you have chosen, it may seem a strange combination, but every birth is different and only fate knows how it will go.

After the birth

The new-born baby will experience the benefit of any remedies that the mother takes, through the breast milk, this should also be kept in mind if taking over the counter drugs, your baby will get a dose too, of just about everything you digest. After the birth, I recommend Rescue Remedy or Star of Bethlehem, especially if there has been trauma, and Walnut, to help the baby make the transition into the world. You can also add the drops to the baby's bath. Bach flowers can be used without any problems in conjunction with homeopathic remedies, as I gave my babies two globules of arnica straight after the birth, and took some myself. I had a wonderful midwife who was experienced with natural birth and homeopathy.

Here is a list of the remedies and their properties, but don't go overboard, try to keep it to a mix of about four or five.

Agrimony - mental torture behind a cheerful face

Aspen - fear of unknown things

Beech - intolerance

Centaury - the inability to say 'no'

Cerato - lack of trust in one's own decisions

Cherry Plum - fear of the mind giving way

Chestnut Bud - failure to learn from mistakes

Chicory - selfish, possessive love

Clematis - dreaming of the future without working in the present

Crab Apple - the cleansing remedy, also for self-hatred

Elm - overwhelmed by responsibility

Gentian - discouragement after a setback

Gorse - hopelessness and despair

Heather - self-centeredness and self-concern

Holly - hatred, envy and jealousy

Honeysuckle - living in the past

Hornbeam - procrastination, tiredness at the thought of doing something

Impatiens - impatience

Larch - lack of confidence

Mimulus - fear of known things

Mustard - deep gloom for no reason

Oak – the mighty oak for physical strength

Olive - exhaustion following mental or physical effort

Pine - guilt

Red Chestnut - over-concern for the welfare of loved ones

Rock Rose - terror and fright

Rock Water - self-denial, rigidity and self-repression

Scleranthus - inability to choose between alternatives

Star of Bethlehem - shock

Sweet Chestnut - Extreme mental anguish, when everything has been tried and there is no light left

Vervain - over-enthusiasm

Vine - dominance and inflexibility

Walnut - protection from change and unwanted influences

Water Violet - pride and aloofness

White Chestnut - unwanted thoughts and mental arguments

Wild Oat - uncertainty over one's direction in life

Wild Rose - drifting, resignation, apathy

Willow - self-pity and resentment

There is also a combination remedy called Rescue Remedy and this is great for calming you down.

Tip

If you're suffering from constipation, why not try making and drinking smoothies. These are like thick fruit juice! Actually they're puréed fruit. Try a half a banana, with a half an apple, half an orange, a quarter mango and if it's too thick, a little more apple juice. A great snack with the plus of fibre.

The second month

This month is especially critical in the development of your baby. Any disturbance from drugs, viruses, or environmental factors such as pesticides may cause birth defects, it is also the most common time for miscarriage. So put on your slippers, put your feet up and relax.

Your baby's development is especially very rapid during the second month. By the end of the second month, all of your baby's major body organs and body systems, including the brain, lungs, liver, and stomach, have begun to develop. The first bone cells appear during this time. Eyelids form and grow but remain closed. The inner ear is forming. Ankles, tiny toes, wrists, fingers, and sexual organs are developing. But you're going to have to wait a while before tickling those toes!

At the end of the second month of pregnancy, your baby looks like a tiny human. If it is a boy, the penis will begin to appear. The baby is a little over 1 inch long and still weighs less than 1 ounce, not a kidney bean anymore! We're getting grape size now! From now on the baby is called a foetus.

I used to have a tiny pin replicate of a pair of feet at eight weeks, it was something I bought to show my feelings against abortion, they were really cute, but got lost over the years.

What is Happening with You

At your prenatal care appointment, your doctor will likely check your weight, your blood pressure, your urine for sugar and protein, and the size of your growing uterus, which is swelling up nicely, even if you can't see it yet. You will also discuss your pregnancy symptoms and any questions you have. It is helpful to write down anything you want to discuss with your doctor, so that you will remember to ask about these things during your appointments, I tend to get very forgetful during pregnancy so I wrote everything down, and just had to remember to take the note with me, but even that often turned out to be too much to remember for me!.

Many women "do not feel pregnant yet" during these early weeks of their pregnancy. This is common, and understandable, you haven't yet got a bump, and you can't feel the baby inside you yet. It is also normal to feel very tired, to urinate often, to feel nausea, to vomit, to have excess saliva, to be constipated, to have heartburn, indigestion, flatulence, or bloating, to experience food aversions or cravings, to feel changes in your breasts (fullness, heaviness, tenderness, tingling, darkening of the areola), to have occasional headaches, to feel faint or dizzy occasionally, and to feel like your clothes are too tight around the waist or boobs. Your emotions are likely to be similar to those you were feeling last month: irritability, mood swings, irrationality, weepiness, misgivings, fear, and happiness. Isn't this getting exciting!

What is Happening with Your Partner

Your partner is also likely to still be feeling a whirlwind of emotions. Remember that is good to talk about how each of is feeling about your pregnancy. Your partner may not know how to help you feel better when you are feeling especially tired, irritable, nauseous, or scared. Talk with each other so that you can work as a team to help you through difficult times.

Your partner may also experience *couvade.* This is a condition that causes the father of the baby to experience weight gain, nausea, mood swings, or other pregnancy symptoms! (Or maybe this could mean your hubby is becoming more empathic!) My husband just put on weight with me, and in some cultures they say if a man puts on weight with his wife, it will be a girl! I say that my constant munching was just contagious! Actually my husband thought my food binges were great, it gave him the excuse to binge with me, but just so I don't feel all alone!

Essential Oils

You may feel nauseous during the first three months of your pregnancy, it's not a very pleasant symptom, but it's reassuring you that your body is doing everything as it should. I found having a bottle of peppermint oil with me at all times very convenient, as it helped me get over the worse of my nausea pangs. Not only peppermint is useful in pregnancy but a whole lot of oils, but remember, only ever use 100% pure essential oils. A lot of people don't know they can use oils during pregnancy, they are afraid it could trigger premature contractions, or harm the baby in some way, and although you should exercise extreme caution, there are some very useful oils to use during this time.

Some discomforts in pregnancy arise from ordinary fluctuations and bodily changes and no matter how uncomfortable they get, always think of them as a reassurance that your body is functioning properly. Some signal a call for dietary or lifestyle adjustments. Most can be eased with the additional use of essential oils.

Aromatherapy is of great help not only in pregnancy, but in preparing the body and mind for pregnancy. As you begin journeying toward the creation of new life, explore the joys of beautifying and caring for yourself. This not only helps you look good, but also helps you feel better about yourself. A lot of women don't feel particularly beautiful during pregnancy, and no matter how much their partner assures them that they are, they just don't feel it. So start pampering yourself and in no time at all, you'll feel truly beautiful, inside and out.

Volatile essential oils extracted from flowers, plants, trees, fruit, and roots provide a natural means of nurturing both body and psyche. Aromatherapy can be used on a regular basis throughout the childbearing year to ease discomforts, alleviate emotional stress, and maintain health and beauty.

Essential Oils for Preconception

Aromatherapy is of great help not only in pregnancy, but in preparing the body and mind for pregnancy. So if you're planning on trying to get pregnant then why not plan some aromatherapy into your routine. Many essential oils are derived from the reproductive apparatus of plants. Flower essences in particular have an alluring aroma that attracts bees, butterflies, and other pollinating creatures. These oils, which are so important to a plants sexuality and reproduction, have physiologic benefits for our own female hormones and reproductive organs. Essential oils from neroli blossom, rose, and jasmine, for example, have numerous yin characteristics, including the ability to calm the nervous system, as well as aphrodisiac qualities and antispasmolytic properties.

The rose is considered the epitome of the feminine. It is associated with the Virgin Mary, who is often depicted with a rose in her hand. Rosaries, from which the Catholic rosary was named, were originally made from dried rosebuds. Hippocrates recommended rose for use in obstetrics. Cleopatra used essence of rose on the sails of her barge to entice the unsuspecting Mark Antony: "The winds were lovesick.... From the barge a strongly invisible perfume hits the sense of the adjacent wharf" (William Shakespeare, Antony and Cleopatra). Sounds like a love spell to me!

In the three months prior to conception, rose essential oil (Rosa damascena), or rose otto, as it is sometimes called, can be of great assistance. Although it is an extremely expensive oil to buy, it goes a long way only needing a tiny bit at a time. To begin with, this oil is known as a fertility promoter. For an increased sperm count, have your partner take warm baths with 4 to 10 drops of rose otto. (Hot baths and hot tubs are to be avoided for three months prior to conception because heat can damage sperm.) Rose oil also helps purify the uterus and regulate the menstrual cycle. To absorb the oil directly into your pelvic region, try sitz baths with 3 to 7 drops of rose otto. More than anything else, rose oil facilitates relaxation and nurtures the emotions. Or even better, bathe together in a bath with rose oil, sprinkled with a few rose petals, a truly romantic evening together.

Partners wishing to nourish each other and strengthen bonds before childbearing can try massaging each other with 4 to 7 drops of rose oil mixed with 1 ounce of carrier oil (grape seed, sweet almond, hazelnut, or other vegetable oil). Other essential oils are also beneficial at this time. Geranium (Pelargonium x asperuin) can help balance the menstrual cycle and hormonal activity. Bergamot (Citrus bergamia), neroli (Citrus aurantium), ylang-ylang (Cananga odorata), and clary sage (Salvia sclarea) are relaxing and uplifting. Maybe I should also mention here that bergamot, and citrus oils can ease winter depression if you suffer from it.

To make a female fertility blend that can counteract the effects of stress, add to 2 ounces of carrier oil: 3 drops of rose, 4 drops of geranium, 3 drops of clary sage, 2 drops of ylang-ylang, and 2 drops of bergamot. A nightly abdominal massage with this blend just before sleep is particularly comforting. Using small, clockwise movements, massage around the entire abdomen, tracing along the inner portion of the pelvic bones, along the diaphragm, and over the solar plexus, then focusing on the lower abdomen in the region of the uterus.

Treating the Discomforts of Pregnancy

Pregnancy can bring on discomforts, and although they are mostly normal, sometimes they are a little less than welcome. Happily most can be eased with the clever use of essential oils.

Nausea, headache, and morning sickness. A woman's sense of smell is heightened during pregnancy you may be intensely attracted to some odours and strongly repelled by others. To keep the atmosphere appealing, use an aromatic diffuser or simply place a few drops of essential oil in a bowl of water so that they can evaporate naturally, scenting the room. The diffuser method, which relies on heat from a candle or an electric bulb, vaporizes the essential oil molecules, spreading the scent faster and farther than the bowl-of-water method. Diffusing antiseptic essential oils into your breathing space will also cleanse the environment of harmful airborne bacteria.

To make a diffuser recipe effective in alleviating morning sickness and headache, mix 3 drops of lavender (Lavendula officinalis or Lavendula vera) with 1 drop of peppermint (Mentha pipperita). If colds or flu are in the air, add 1 drop of eucalyptus (Eucalyptus globulus) as a preventative.

To help combat nausea, place a cool lavender oil compress on your forehead and a warm lavender oil compress over the front of your rib cage. A deep whiff of peppermint oil will often cure nausea, as will a cup of tea or honey water prepared with 1 drop of peppermint oil. (Do not overuse peppermint, as it can have stimulating effects, and do not take essential oils internally on an empty stomach.

Lavender and peppermint are good remedies for headaches as well. At the first sign of headache, place 1 drop of undiluted lavender oil on each temple, or lying down in a dimly lit room, place a cool peppermint oil compress on your forehead. To counteract strange or bad odours when out and about, keep a cotton hankie dabbed with 1 drop of lavender or peppermint oil in a plastic bag in your purse. To prevent headache or nausea, hold the hankie over your nose and inhale deeply; repeat as necessary.

Morning sickness often occurs during the third month of pregnancy, usually in response to the sitting of the placenta. It can also arise in response to low blood sugar levels after a night of fasting, meaning a few hours without food! Nutritionists recommend a healthy, protein-rich snack along with carbohydrates and fruit before bed and again in the morning before getting up. Morning sickness can also result from a vitamin B-6 deficiency.

To help vomiting, or rather to ease it add 7 drops of lemon (Citrus limon) or lavender oil to 1 ounce of carrier oil, and massage over the abdomen--or simply inhale the essences. A cup of red raspberry leaf (Rubus strigosus) tea can provide relief while toning the uterus, this tea is well known to be useful during pregnancy. If morning sickness is severe, try tincture of wild yam root (Dioscorea villosa); add the extract to boiling water or hot tea as recommended on the label.

Legal ailments and haemorrhoids. Weight gain and abdominal pressure due to increased blood volume and the softening effects of progesterone on the venous walls may cause varicose veins, oedema, other leg discomforts and haemorrhoids, particularly in the second trimester. Leg discomforts during pregnancy are also attributed to nutrient deficiencies, and of course you're carrying a lot more weight around than you're used to. A boost in vitamin B-6 is often recommended for varicose veins, oedema, and leg cramps. Vitamin E helps prevent varicose veins and blood clots. Garlic cleanses the circulatory system. Sodium helps alleviate leg cramps, as does calcium, or magnesium.

Varicose veins respond well to the toning and astringent properties of cypress (Cupressus sempervirens), geranium, lemon, and lavender oils. Elevating your legs, alternating warm and cool compresses of any combination of these oils to the affected area can help. Bathe in warm water mixed with 3 drops of cypress and 3 drops of lemon. Using a blend of 7 drops of cypress and 7 drops of lemon mixed with 2 ounces of carrier oil, gently stroke from the feet upward. While massaging, be careful not to apply strong pressure over a varicosity or just below the point at which a varicosity begins.

Oedema (fluid retention) of the ankles or legs responds to lavender, geranium, and rosemary (Rosmarinus officinalis) oils, all of which stimulate the lymphatic system to drain excess fluids from the body, although I ate a lot of potatoes with the skins to help this. Using upward strokes, gently massage a blend of these oils to the feet and ankles. If your feet are hot, tired, or swollen, try tepid-to-cool footbaths with 3 drops of geranium or lemon and 3 drops of lavender. To reduce swelling, sleep with a pillow under your legs, and take afternoon naps with your legs elevated higher than your heart. To strengthen the venous walls, add vitamin C and buckwheat to your diet. Exercise, especially walking and swimming, will stimulate circulation, as will support tights worn on a regular basis. Baths with lemon, mandarin (Citrus reticulata), or other citrus oils contain vitamin C and will provide a mild diuretic action.

Dilated veins that cause swollen anal tissue result from the same conditions that cause varicose veins; they're also a result from repeated straining to pass stool. The herb nettle leaf (Urtica dioica) can be taken as an infusion or tincture to improve elasticity of the veins and reduce haemorrhoids. Also add oat bran to your breakfast cereal, and be sure to eat plenty of fruit and vegetables. Cool sitz baths with 7 drops of lemon oil will help, as will a follow-up massage using 7 drops of cypress plus 7 drops of lemon oil in 2 ounces of carrier oil.

Insomnia and Nightmares

Comfortable sleeping positions can be hard to find in the later stages of pregnancy. If you are having trouble getting to sleep, or staying asleep, try lying on your left side with a pillow between your knees and additional pillows supporting your arms and back. Sprinkle neroli blossom or sandalwood (Santalum album) oil around your bed, or dot a drop or two on your pillow. These oils, soothing to the mind and emotions, act as sedatives to relieve anxiety; their fragrant aromas will help you drift easily off to sleep. Also try sprinkling a few drops of essential oil in a bowl of water near a radiator or heat vent. A warm neroli oil bath before bed can help relieve the day's stress and invite a sound sleep. If muscle cramps are keeping you awake, take a calcium-magnesium supplement before retiring, or as my mom used to, drink a warm cocoa, the milk contains calcium and magnesium, these relax the body, and real cocoa contains Tryptophan, a chemical that the brain uses to make a neurotransmitter called serotonin. High levels of serotonin can produce feelings of elation, it also contains phenyl ethylamine and Anandamide, both these chemicals make a person happy, and if your guilty conscience screams “too many calories” here’s a bit of trivia for you.....

Researchers at Harvard University have carried out experiments that suggest that if you eat chocolate three times a month you will live almost a year longer than those who forego such sweet temptation. (This must mean I’ll live to be a hundred and fifty!!)

Antioxidants; Cocoa beans contain polyphenols (similar to those found in wine) with antioxidant properties which are health beneficial. These compounds are called flavonoids and include catechins, epicatechins, and procyandins. The antioxidant flavinoids are found in the non-fat portions of the cocoa bean. The flavinoids also reduce the blood's ability to clot and thus reduces the risk of stroke and heart attacks.

Phenyl ethylamine; Phenyl ethylamine is a slight antidepressant and stimulant similar to the body's own dopamine and adrenaline.

Serotonin; Cocoa and chocolate can increase the level of serotonin in the brain. Serotonin levels are often decreased in people with depression and in those experiencing PMS symptoms.

Essential minerals; Cocoa beans are rich in a number of essential minerals, including magnesium, calcium, iron, zinc, copper, potassium and manganese.

Vitamins; A, B1, B2, B3, C, E and pantothenic acid.

So there you go, helps to ease you off to sleep, and is good for you!

Back to pregnancy problems....Pregnant women's nightmares about themselves or their babies are considered a normal release of anxiety about parenthood and the well-being of the child. The remedy of choice is essential oil of frankincense (Boswellia carterii). Sprinkle it around your bed, place a drop or two on your pillow, put a few drops in a bowl of water near a heat source, or massage your chest with 1 drop of frankincense mixed with 1 teaspoon of carrier oil. Applied to the back of the neck, this oil is said to be especially protective. A cup of tea made with skullcap (Scutellaria lateriflora) extract soothes raw nerves and restores deep sleep.

Stretch Marks

Most women fear these more than the flabby thighs, as even after the birth, though they fade, a pale silver mark always remains. They cannot be "cured", never fading completely, so they must be prevented. To prevent stretch marks and keep your skin soft and supple, use topical applications of vegetable oils. To maintain elasticity, stock up on vitamins C and E. Evening primrose oil capsules, taken internally, also nourish the skin and help maintain elasticity, my midwife told me to take a combination of evening primrose and borage after the thirteenth week to help prepare the cervix and soften the os (cervic mouth), rubbed on to the perinea, it will make it more elastic and the use of Episiotomy is reduced, you can literally insert two capsules into the vagina before going to bed. They will melt during the night. Wheat germ oil, applied topically, is a wonderful stretch mark preventative, for it neutralizes acidity and toxins and is a natural source of vitamin E. Hazelnut oil is similarly rich in vitamin E.

To make a stretch mark blend, mix 1 ounce of hazelnut oil and 1 ounce of wheat germ oil with 4 drops of neroli, 2 drops of carrot seed (Daucus carota), and 2 drops of geranium oil. Morning and evening, massage this blend into thighs, hips, breasts, and belly. Or add the blend to warm bathwater mixed with seaweed extract or seawater concentrate for a mineralizing soak. To avoid dehydrating your skin, do not take overly hot baths and do not soap up your entire body after emerging from the tub, pat off excess water with a towel, leaving the skin damp. Then apply stretch mark blend and body lotion.

Chloasma

The so-called mask of pregnancy (hyper pigmentation), sounds scary...it has been linked to the inability of the liver to remove excess hormones from the bloodstream. Pigmentation problems also result from a deficiency of folic acid, PABA, vitamin B-12, or vitamin B-6. To protect your skin from sunlight, wear sunscreen and a hat. At night, apply several drops of the following essential oil blend to your facial skin: 3 drops of lemon plus 4 drops of myrtle (Myrtus communis) to 1 ounce of carrier oil. Work the blend into your skin with cool water or floral water. Then apply your preferred face cream.

Acne

Some women say that their skin never looked better than when they were pregnant, they get a real glow that my mom always calls the look of pregnancy. Others prone to the surging hormonal activity of pregnancy say the opposite. If you are among those subject to acne, dab on a tiny amount of undiluted lavender oil. For an inflamed pustule, use 1 drop of tea tree oil (Maleleuca alternafolia). A weekly mask of seaweed extracts and mineral-rich clay will help keep skin clear of dead cells and debris.

Essential Oil Massage for Pregnancy

Touch is a profound part of your sensory experience. A daily massage can activate millions of nerve receptors, regulate and balance bodily functions, and send a message of love and care to your baby. Self-massage is one approach; massage by your partner is another. Massage is a lovely way for fathers to be involved in pregnancy and to get to know their babies.

Care of the perineum

Much can be done during pregnancy to prepare the perineum to stretch beyond its everyday limits for birth, and to do so without tearing and without the need for surgical cutting. Midwives who incorporate aromatherapy into their practice have found that episiotomy or tearing occurs in only 48 percent of birthing women who perform perinea massage during pregnancy, compared with 77 percent of those who do not. I gave you one of the remedies I got from my midwife above, here's another way to massage the perineum using essential oils, or you can use the evening primrose and borage oil. I wanted to avoid an episiotomy at all costs, I find it unnatural and an intrusion.

Massage your perineum for 5 to 10 minutes a day beginning five or six weeks before your due date. First, empty your bladder. Follow with a 5- to 15-minute warm water and lavender oil, sitz bath to relax the vaginal wall. Then, inserting two well-washed index fingers or thumbs into the vagina just enough to stretch the perinea tissue, press the vaginal wall back toward the rectum. Massaging in a U-shaped motion with a blend of 3 drops of lavender, 1 drop of geranium, and 1 ounce of wheat germ oil, stretch the vagina open for 20 to 60 seconds, or until you feel a tingling or slight burning sensation-precisely what you will feel with the crowning of baby's head in labour. Over time, the perinea tissue will become soft and supple.

With daily massages of this sort, the perineum is likely to remain highly elastic and intact during birth. If tearing should occur, or if an episiotomy becomes necessary, treat yourself to warm postpartum baths or sitz baths to speed the healing. Add cypress, lavender, or geranium oil to the bathwater to help tighten the stretched or severed tissue, prevent infection, and stop the bleeding. For an effective soak, use 3 drops of cypress and 3 drops of lavender.

I'd like to add here that I did avoid an episiotomy on all three of my deliveries. My third delivery went so smooth and I had prepared so well, that immediately after the birth my midwife commented that she had never seen the like of it before, you would never guess that a baby had just passed through my birth canal, not even a single bruise.

Care of the full body

Treat every part of your body to an essential oil massage, especially in the later months of pregnancy. A foot massage is a wonderful way to enliven the entire body and relieve the legs of pressure. To position yourself for massage of the back and neck, sit backward on a straight-backed chair, or sit on a stool and lean forward onto a table piled with pillows for support. Reclining, prop yourself up with cushions and pillows for massage of the neck, back, shoulders, and limbs. And remember, massage of the abdomen calls for the lightest of strokes.

Essential Oils for Labour and Birth

Aromatherapy, increasingly endorsed by midwives throughout the world, is slowly gaining acceptance in hospitals throughout Europe and the United Kingdom. German midwife trainees are required to study aromatherapy as part of their course curriculum, and in Switzerland most birthing houses would use it for all births. Indeed, monitoring equipment has shown that foetal heartbeat variability accompanying foetal distress can be normalized when mothers are given an essential oil body massage. And I was lucky to receive aromatherapy massages for my births. I can honestly say it was wonderful.

Plan on creating a magical birthing environment, complete with soft lights, music, and your favourite essential oils. Neroli, bergamot, rose, and frankincense can help relieve anxiety and fears you might be harbouring about birth. Breathing in any of these oils as they waft through the air from your diffuser will help you relax between contractions, inviting your body's production of endorphins to provide natural pain relief. Simply add to the diffuser 3 or 4 drops of your chosen oil.

Lavender (Lavendula augustifolia) can promote relaxation and pain relief during labour. Once your contractions are established and your cervix has dilated at least 2 centimetres, plan on taking a long lavender soak. Women who bathe for 30 minutes or more during this phase of labour experience improved progress and a significant decrease in the need for drugs.

An essential oil massage between contractions can be soothing and comforting while stimulating pain relief. A foot massage may be ideal, or perhaps a low back massage with gentle, yet firm strokes, using the palm of the hand. For a top-notch labour blend, combine 20 drops of lavender and 8 drops of clary sage in 4 ounces of carrier oil.

To help stimulate and strengthen contractions, request a jasmine (Iasminum grandiflorum) compress on the lower abdomen or sacrum, although a pricey compress, it does work wonders. For pain, use lavender or clary sage. Cool compresses to the forehead can help ward off fatigue and keep you refreshed. If nausea crops up, take a whiff of peppermint or lavender.

Spikenard (Nardostachys jatamansi), an exotic essential oil not often mentioned in aromatherapy literature, is profoundly relaxing. Spikenard's sedative action is useful if pain and tension are keeping you from opening into your contractions. In such instances, be sure to ask for an abdominal massage with 8 drops of spikenard mixed with 7 drops of jasmine and 3 drops of lemon verbena in 4 ounces of carrier oil. Or apply a compress of this blend just above the pubic hair. Evening primrose oil can be massaged directly on the cervix if it remains rigid and non-dilating.

Labour is a wondrous act of nature, and unique to every childbearing woman. If pain or tension gets you down, remember that this stage will pass. Envision yourself as a powerful woman, research which goddess you could call upon to help you through, and know that in a very short time, you will be holding your baby in your arms. Try to remember, the sensation you register as pain, is just the effort your body is making to bring your baby into this world, try not to think of it as pain as such. Knowledge is definitely power here!

Quality and Safety Guidelines

Ask questions and be discriminating when selecting essential oils. Purchase only those that have been distilled for therapeutic use. Such oils are termed "genuine," "authentic," or "of therapeutic quality." Check to see that the oils you buy are of the botanical species noted in the text, are unadulterated (free of additives, even natural ones), are not deterpenated (subjected to laboratory removal of terpenes), and are steam distilled under pressure to ensure the completeness of their components. High-quality essential oils are tested by gas chromatograph to assess their chemical constituents and to detect adulterants. Unfortunately, many of the essential oils available today are of a lesser grade, and are not suitable for healing purposes.

Certain essential oils are emmenagogic (bringing on menstruation) and are subject to controversy. Some texts list them as unsafe in pregnancy, whereas others point out that they are wonderful for pregnancy. The following essential oils are emmenagogic: caraway, cedar wood, chamomile, clary sage, cypress, jasmine, juniper, lavender, marjoram, nutmeg, peppermint, rose, and rosemary. So use sparingly.

Certain essential oils are known abortifacients and are to be avoided during pregnancy These include: ajowan, aniseed, basil, bitter almond, boldo, buchu, camphor, dove, cornmint, cotton lavender, fennel, horseradish, hyssop, lavendula stoechas, mugwort, mustard, myrrh, oregano, parsley seed, pennyroyal--American and European, pimenta racemosa, plecanthrus, rue, sage (not to be confused with clary sage), sassafras, savin, savory, star anise, sweet birch, sweet marjoram, tansy, tarragon, thuja, thyme (C.T. thymol), West Indian. bay leaf, wild thyme, wintergreen, wormseed, and wormwood.

Methods and Dosages

Massage blends

The maximum dosage for use in pregnancy is a 1 percent dilution. To prepare a 1 percent dilution, add 10 to 14 drops of essential oil to 2 ounces of carrier oil, or add 5 to 7 drops of essential oil to 1 ounce of carrier oil. Two percent dilutions are suitable for use before and after pregnancy. Never use undiluted essential oils directly on your skin unless specifically recommended.

Baths and sitz baths

Use a maximum of 6 drops of essential oil per bath. To prepare a sitz bath, set a large plastic baby tub in your bathtub, fill with water, add the oils, and agitate to spread. Lower yourself into the baby tub, keeping your feet on the outside, and soak for 20 minutes unless otherwise directed. An aromatherapy bath in the morning can prepare you for a smooth and easy-to-cope-with-stress day. To eliminate the urge for caffeine, try an uplifting oil such as lemon or geranium oil. An evening bath with relaxing oils such as sandalwood or frankincense can soak away the day's troubles and calm the nervous system for a sound sleep.

Compresses

Fill a bowl with cool or warm water, depending on your needs. Add 3 or 4 drops of essential oil. For cool compresses, drape a flannel across the top of the cool water to pick up a film of the oil, then wring out the flannel and place it on the appropriate body area; repeat when the compress has warmed. For warm compresses, drape the flannel, wring it out, place it on the body, and cover it with plastic and a towel; repeat when the compress has cooled.

Inhalations

For a diffuser, use 3 to 4 drops of essential oil. For a hankie, use 1 drop.

Tip

If your nausea is bad, try peppermint oil on a hanky, take a whiff every now and then, and of course Ginger ale! But it must have real ginger extract. Having dry crackers on your bedside table is also handy, eat one before you stand up, works wonders!

The Third month

Your baby will be completely formed by the end of the third month. Your baby may have begun moving its hands, legs, and head and opening and closing its mouth, but he or she is still too small for you to feel this movement, unless you meditate often, in which, you may be more aware of changes in your body, although the earliest I felt a baby was on my second pregnancy with my daughter, at sixteen weeks during meditation I felt like a tapping sensation, but the doctor didn't believe me saying it was too early, although my midwife did, she said it is rare but some women are more in tune with the baby.

The fingers and toes are now more distinct and have soft nails. The baby's hands are more developed than the feet and the arms are longer than the legs. Your baby's head is quite large compared to the rest of its body. Hair may have started to form on the head. Tooth buds have formed under the baby's gums. Vocal cords develop around the 13th week of pregnancy, although junior will have to wait a bit to use them!.

Your baby's heart has four chambers and beats at 120 to 160 beats per minute. Kidneys are now developed and start draining urine into the bladder. Intestines have formed outside of the baby (on the umbilical cord) because they can't fit inside the baby. By the end of this month, the umbilical cord, which carries nutrients to your baby and takes wastes away, will be fully formed.

At the end of your third month, your baby will weigh just over 1 ounce and will be about 4 inches long, he or she could nestle comfortably into a tea cup.

What is Happening with You

At your prenatal care appointment this month, your doctor will again check your weight, blood pressure, and urine. In addition, your doctor will likely check the foetal heartbeat, the size of the uterus to see how it correlates with the estimated due date, and the height of the fundus (the top of the uterus). Remember to bring any questions and concerns you and your partner may have so that you can discuss them with your doctor.

Many of the early physical pregnancy symptoms continue during the third month. However, you may begin to notice additional veins appearing on your breasts, abdomen, legs, and elsewhere as the blood supply increases. Your abdomen may appear larger by the end of this month. Your appetite is likely to increase. For some women this is getting exciting, they finally have a belly to show!

Your emotions may continue to switch back and forth between happiness, fear, joy, misgivings and you may still feel somewhat unstable. However, many women begin to experience a new sense of calmness around this time. You may also be offered you first ultra scan, this is for some women, me included really exciting, seeing your baby move on the screen is a wonderful feeling and for fathers who find it hard to realise that their partner is carrying life inside her, the proof. My husband cried the first time he watched our son on the screen. He went out and bought a rocking horse the next day!

What is Happening with Your Partner

Other than the fact that he might suddenly feel the urge to buy a rocking horse! Only kidding! He might start to get excited now too, especially if your belly is starting to swell. Involve your partner in your pregnancy by discussing your emotions together, see if he has any questions for your doctor, and share books and videos you are using to learn more about how to take care of yourself and your baby.

Herbals

The Pregnancy Tea

Equal parts of

Meadowsweet (which is often referred to as 'nature's tums' and is nature's gift to the pregnant woman)

Chamomile (which has been shown to have a soothing and healing effect and tastes wonderful)

Raspberry Leaf (this is truly the woman's herb, used all over the world by pregnant women, prepares the womb for birth by relaxing and strengthening the uterus, smoothes menstrual cycle, helps nausea, other GI upsets)

Plus a bit of

Hops (calming, also particularly good for insomnia, tension)

Marshmallow root (a great demulcent, coats gastro-intestinal tract)

Nettle (strengthens and nourishes, iron, vitamin C, also helps increase milk production in nursing mothers)

Lemon Balm (great for flavour, combines well with nettle and raspberry leaf in women's formulas)

Peppermint/Spearmint (wonderful for upset stomach of any kind, stimulates release of stomach acids, use large amounts for fevers and flues, generally soothing).

Not all of these must be used for the tea to be productive. However, the Chamomile, Raspberry Leaf, and Meadowsweet are the most important and I must strongly encourage the use of a mint. It is a nice idea to buy a bit of each herb (find a store that sells bulk by weight- it's not as expensive as you'd think) and to combine them and store them in a sealable jar. It is much more convenient than mixing it each time. But it is nice to experiment in the beginning and invent a tea to best suit your individual needs and tastes. This is only what worked the best for me.

Herbs to avoid during pregnancy: Goldenseal, Mandrake, Mugwort, Tansy, Rue, Wormwood (which tastes awful in any way), Barberry, Horsetail, Cohosh, Ginger (except in small doses)*,

Hyssop, Motherwort, Myrrh, Parsley, Pennyroyal, Sage, Shepard's Purse, Liquorice, Dong Quai, Ginseng, Sarsaparilla.

*Ginger may be used in small amounts during pregnancy in recipes or to help relieve heartburn symptoms. Just be sure to follow directions carefully and not to overdo it!

And during the last two to four weeks, a tea can be drunk to help prepare you for birth and to help avoid going over your date!

One litre of water, bring to the boil with;

Half a cinnamon stick

Ten cloves

Tablespoon of verbena

Turn off the heat and let it seep for ten minutes before straining.

The Fourth Month

The baby's skin is pink and somewhat transparent. Eyebrows and eyelashes begin to appear in this month. Buds on the side of the head begin to form into the outer ear. The baby's face continues to develop. The tail has disappeared from the foetus and the head makes up about half of the baby's size. The baby's neck is long enough to lift the head from the body. And looking so cute now!

The baby moves, kicks, sleeps, wakes, swallows, and passes urine. You may start to feel a slight sensation in your lower abdomen (called quickening). This feels like bubbles or fluttering.

When you feel the baby's movement, this is a magical experience for all mothers, the first real movement! Write down the date and tell your health care provider. This helps determine when your baby is due. This will cause you to become very excited and although impossible for an outside person to feel, you should still feel free to pester your partner to keep feeling and waiting for a flutter!

By the end of the fourth month, your baby will be 8 to 10 inches long and will weigh about 6 ounces. I think we need a bigger tea cup!

What is Happening with You

During prenatal care appointments in the fourth

month, your doctor will likely check your weight, blood pressure, urine, foetal heartbeat, size of your uterus, height of your fundus, any swelling or varicose veins, and other symptoms. It is important to continue to monitor all of these continually during your pregnancy to help ensure the health of your baby and prevent or lessen any problems you might experience.

This is the month that many women start to "feel pregnant." Physically, you may still be fatigued, feel constipated, have indigestion, heartburn, flatulence, or bloating, and experience occasional headaches and dizziness. Some of the symptoms you may have had during the first trimester will likely decrease or go away. For example, you will not need to urinate as frequently, what a relief! You can make it to the local shop and back without stopping for a pee! You will feel less nauseated and be less likely to vomit, and your breasts will not feel as tender but will continue to grow. New symptoms that you may experience include: nasal congestion and occasional nosebleeds, ear stuffiness, bleeding gums, increase in your appetite, mild swelling in your ankles, feet, hands, and face, varicose veins in your legs and/or haemorrhoids, a slight whitish vaginal discharge (leucorrhoea), clumsiness, and possibly foetal movement toward the end of the month. Remember that all women experience pregnancy differently and you may have none, some, or all of these symptoms.

Your emotions are likely to still swing back and forth between joy, apprehension, irritability, etc. Many women feel frustrated and self-conscious about their bodies when they don't fit into their regular clothes but are still too small for maternity clothes. You may also feel somewhat scattered and clumsy--it is normal to be forgetful, drop things, and have trouble concentrating. (I can assure you, it will return to normal after the birth! or at least after junior starts sleeping)

What is Happening with Your Partner

Your partner may now be worrying mostly about money at this point. And not because you're eating him into poverty! Worrying will cause unnecessary stress and irritability in both you and your partner. The money will work out when the baby comes. You can both work together on trying to save money now. However, this is not the time to become stressed about how you will put your as yet unborn child through college. But men being men will worry, it gives them something to do while you're busy being clumsy!!

You both will probably want to continue to read or watch videos about pregnancy and newborn care. Check out pregnancy and childbirth classes near you and find out how soon you need to register for them. These classes often fill up quickly. Many of them are appropriate for both you and your partner. Although I never attended one, I have friends who say they are really worthwhile, I was of the opinion my body knows better, and I concentrated on keeping my mind fit, as I was planning on a birth without medical interference, and courses just seemed too unnatural for me, maybe if there was a pagan course I would have went.

If you're planning on having your baby in a hospital, you could take a tour of the labour ward, this is a great chance to ask questions about how everything runs in the hospital. It was after three of these tours in different hospitals that I decided I was going to give birth in a birthing house, I didn't like the idea of not having complete control over my birth.

Reflexology

Many people have heard of Reflexology and know of its many successes, and its ability to restore balance when this has been undermined by disorders and ill health, but did you know that it can also be of benefit to the healthy mother-to-be during pregnancy and childbirth?

Reflexology treatment trials carried out on pregnant mothers to help control high blood pressure not only reduced the amount of hospital admissions for the patients but it was also discovered that these women had really easy births. This work was pioneered by Dr. Gowri Motha, a gynaecologist, who happens to train many reflexologists and midwives in the care and treatment of mothers-to-be during pregnancy and childbirth.

As well as helping with all the normal effects of pregnancy like nausea and vomiting, reflexology treatment encourages the uterus to become a very healthy muscle. The pelvis may flare more easily and the cervix may dilate more rapidly. As yet, we do not know exactly what initiate's labour, but a pacemaker area within the uterus opens up the cervix. This coupled with pressure from the baby's head co-ordinate uterine action.

It is normally recommended that where the mother-to-be has not received reflexology previously, that she wait for week eighteen before commencing treatment. If previous treatment has been given, then it should be safe to have treatment from conception. It is helpful if treatment is performed fortnightly up until week 38. This can be stepped up if specific problems like backache or high blood pressure arise.

Perhaps no mother-to-be needs reminding to eat well and exercise during pregnancy... but ballet, aerobics, belly dancing and horse riding are not good to do as the muscles become hard and may delay the birth, your body starts relaxing the joints and bones during pregnancy, and this also makes backache and other symptoms more pronounced. Although belly dancing would probably look very interesting at this time!

Reflexology will aid pregnancy by stimulating the liver, endocrine (hormone releasing) glands and lymphatic drainage. Attention is of course paid to the pelvic and reproductive areas. Apparently, pregnancies do tend to go to term with reflexology.

Quite importantly, reflexology can be performed prior to conception, particularly where there is a history of miscarriage. It has also been noted that babies whose mothers have received preconceptual treatment are seldom bad tempered. No comment!

When medical conditions such as septicaemia are present then treatment is contra-indicated and any unusual effects like vaginal bleeding must be referred for medical attention. Having said this, there does seem to be less need for medical intervention when reflexology has been performed.

If all is going well, it is quite in order to have treatment during the early stages of labour and currently more hospitals have a policy of allowing access to complementary practitioners. This would of course need discussing with your medical team during pregnancy.

Remember that visualisation can be of extraordinary help and visualising a fast and easy delivery can work wonders.

Dream Catcher

Wouldn't it be a nice Idea to make a dream catcher for baby's room? All my kids have one in their room, and they all have little charms attached to them to make them extra special too.

Making a dream catcher is fairly easy, and fun to do. It's a way to spend time concentrating on your baby before it is born. Here's how you make one!

Materials:

Thin, round, basket-weaving reed - (This can be purchased at an arts and craft store.)

String or twine

Beads, feathers

Yarn

Directions:

Step 1: Take a length of reed equivalent to approximately 26 inches, form into a circle and secure by overlapping and bending the two loose ends around the edge of the circle. The circle width should be 5 to 5 1/2 inches, of course you can make the dream catcher any size you wish. To strengthen the circle and prevent it from coming undone, you may tightly wrap the entire circle with a length of colourful yarn.

Step 2: To begin making the dream catcher "web," tie one end of the twine or string to the circle you have formed in step one. Tie 9 "hitch knots" around the ring, spacing them approximately 2 inches apart. Keep the string snug when going from one knot to the next being careful not to distort the shape of the circle. See diagram below:

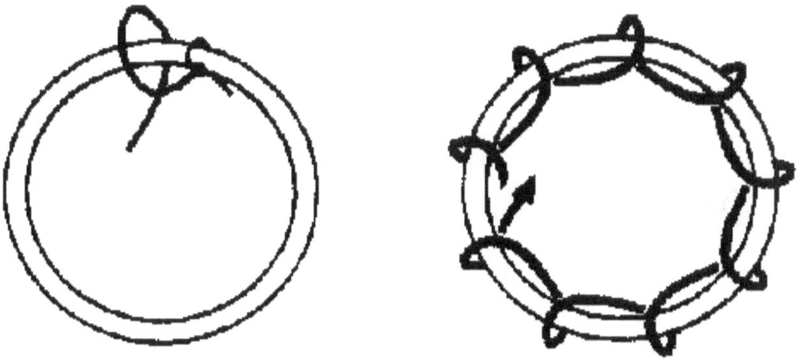

Step 3: To begin the next row of the web, begin tying hitch knots in the middle of the string already attached. Continue tying hitches in the same way until the opening in the centre is the desired size. To end the web, tie a double knot in the twine and cut off any excess. See diagram below:

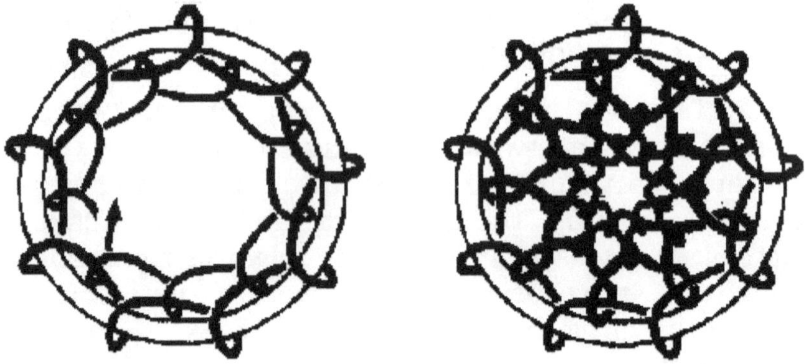

Step 4: To decorate the dream catcher: Each student will need about 2 feet of string for attaching beads and/or feathers. Cut string into 4 equal pieces and thread the beads or tie the feathers to the ends. Tie these decorate strings to the bottom, sides, and centre of the dream catcher. Be sure to attach a hanging loop to the top.

The Fifth Month

Your belly will be swelling nicely now, my mom always said at this time the pregnant woman starts to bloom. Your baby is growing rapidly at this time. The internal organs are maturing. Your baby's fingernails have grown to the tips of the fingers. Fat is now being stored beneath your baby's skin. Your baby is also growing muscle and is getting stronger every day, those little jabs are making themselves noticed. The blood cells take over for the liver the job of producing blood. Your baby's gall bladder will start working, producing bile that is necessary for digestion. Milk teeth will begin forming under your baby's gums. Body hair, including eyebrows and eyelashes, are starting to grow.

Your baby sleeps and wakes at regular intervals. You will find that your baby is much more active now. He or she turns from side to side and head over heels. Your baby may suck its thumb, a habit that sometimes last past birth.

At the end of the fifth month, your baby will be about 10-12 inches long and will weigh about 1 pound, that's a bag of sugar!

What is Happening with You

Your doctor will again check your weight, blood pressure, urine, foetal heartbeat, uterus size, fundal height, and check for any swelling in hands and feet, varicose veins and haemorrhoids, or any other symptoms you may be experiencing.

Remember to bring your list of questions and concerns with you to your prenatal care appointments so that you can discuss them with your doctor.

You may be experiencing any number of the following physical symptoms: foetal movement, increasing whitish vaginal discharge (leucorrhoea), lower abdomen achiness (from stretching of the ligaments which support the uterus), constipation, heartburn, indigestion, flatulence, or bloating, occasional headaches, faintness, or dizziness, nasal congestion, nosebleeds, ear stuffiness, bleeding gums, hearty appetite, leg cramps, swelling, varicose veins, haemorrhoids, increased heart rate, backache, and/or changes in your skin pigmentation of your abdomen and face. Remember that you may not feel all of these symptoms. The palms of my hands always went reddish during pregnancy, and because I have very pale skin, I always thought it looked funny, but nobody else ever noticed it.

Your emotions are probably calming down now and you are likely to have fewer mood swings. You may still feel irritable from time to time. Absentmindedness and forgetfulness may still continue, I call this constant readiness for meditation! Only kidding.

If you are planning on having a home birth or a birth in a birthing house, you may now start having regular appointments with your midwife, I feel it makes a really big difference in how the birth goes if you have a friendly relationship with the midwife who is delivering your baby, and you are more likely to be open about how you feel during the birth, not to mention there will be no doctors buzzing in and out of the room. But if you are considering one of these options you must be clear that there will be no painkillers available to you should you want them, such births are natural, and will lean more to homeopathy, aromatherapy and touch therapy (massage etc.) And personally, a natural birth is more magical than the average controlled hospital birth. But saying that, a lot of hospitals are becoming more open to natural births, and are happy to make a compromise when it comes to monitoring machines and drips etc.

What is Happening with Your Partner

Your partner is probably enjoying that you are feeling calmer and are having fewer mood swings! It is still important to communicate how you are both feeling. You may welcome it if your partner wants to "baby" and take care of you during your pregnancy or you may resent it. If your partner wants to baby you or help around the house, let him. It's his way of showing you how excited or happy he is.

If you decide like I had to not go to a hospital to give birth, your partner may feel apprehensive, my husband was told by a lot of his friends to force me to be in a hospital in case anything went wrong, but he knows how I am and respected that, as I would be taking more of an active role in the birth as he would be (literally), that the decision would be mine. He also trusted the midwife that if anything went wrong, I would be in the hospital within ten minutes.

Remember to sign up for pregnancy and childbirth classes that you can both attend. And maybe visit a birth house together.

Aura Soma

In 1984 the name Aura-Soma and the vision of its creation, was bestowed upon its chosen custodian - Vicky Wall. Vicky claims she received visions containing the same message repeatedly - she was told to 'go and divide the waters, My Child'.

Vicky, a practicing chiropodist, pharmacist and herbalist was 66 years of age and 'clinically' blind at the time. She had no idea what she was doing that night when she was impulsed to go to her small laboratory and formulate a mixture comprising of different layers and colours of natural ingredients.

'Equilibrium' was born that night. Vicky later reported that "other hands had guided her own' - for she could neither 'see' the beautiful jewels she had spontaneously and inspirationally created, or their possible intended purpose. Even more bewildering, was the resonant power she felt emanating from them, as they basked in the sunlight of the following morning, clearly revealing two distinctly separate and different layers.

Thousands of Vicky's' clients were attracted to the 'Equilibrium' Bottles and this allowed her to build a formal body of solidly researched scientific knowledge.

Why did people spontaneously choose certain bottles? What affect did the bottle/s have on their life after continued exposure to it/them? What were the individuals 'life dynamics' before and after continued exposure to or use of the contents of certain bottles?

Over a period of a few short years, this scientific approach verified the answers to all these questions and more. With absolute certainty Vicky was able to verify the premise that 'Colour speaks a language of its own.'

What is aura soma?

The Language of Colour: Aura-Soma is an ancient Knowledge Trust reborn. This Trust is being shared at this pivotal point in Earth history in the universal language that every HUE-MAN has inherently understood since the Creator said, 'Let There Be Light'. That is ... 'The Language of Colour'.

This 'Window of the Soul' reveals our most deeply hidden aspects in a form that we can understand, embrace, accept and otherwise grow through. It has often been stated of Aura-Soma, 'You are the colours you choose" and that these colours not only metaphor your true being, but facilitate communication between self and Soul via 'The Rainbow Bridge'. I have to say it can be very interesting to sit in front of the bright lit displays of colourful bottles and choose one to later read what it means.

This 'Living Energy' is the heart of Aura-Soma. Its ability to gently guide and reward us with a richly deep understanding and experience of ourselves and the future we are co-creating is absolutely profound. The word Aura comes from the Latin meaning: akin to air, a slight breath, vapour or shimmer. Soma is the ancient Greek word for 'body', while in ancient Sanskrit it designates a mysterious drink that transports the soul into a Divine ecstasy.

When the two words are combined, they set up a very different and specific vibration, as both concepts; Aura and Soma have essentially deeper meaning inherent in them.

In the equilibrium there are special sets for special purposes, one being the New Aeon Child set, with the bottles numbered, eleven, twelve, thirteen, fourteen, and fifteen.

The New Aeon Child Set is meant to accompany a child from birth, and to support him/her until he/she becomes a responsible young adult.

Bottle #11 can also be used by a couple desiring to conceive a child, as Clear/Pink supports a "conscious conception". This Set brings many benefits to both the mother and the unborn child during pregnancy, with #12, #13, and #14, being used for as many days, weeks or months as the intuition of the mother indicates is right.

A Chain of Flowers

Bottle #11 Clear/Pink

Bottle #11 is suitable for use on newborn children, and should be continued until either nine months of age or until the fontanels close. #11 is also very helpful with ear infections in children - regardless of the age.

Peace in the new Aeon

Bottle #12 Clear/Blue

#12 should be used until the end of the nursing period. If the child is not nursed, then use should continue until he/she can drink out of a cup by themselves. If this transition has proven difficult, then the Clear/Blue Oil will ease the transition

Change in the new Aeon

Bottle #13 Clear/Green

Bottle #13 should be used on the child until the "rebellious" phase - often referred to as the "terrible twos" is over. Continuous use of the Clear/Green Oil will soften this phase

Wisdom in the new Aeon

Bottle #14 Clear/Gold

#14 should be used until the beginning of school - around age 6 or 7. As its' name implies, it opens the way to subtle inner wisdom that otherwise would be difficult to access and integrate.

Healing in the new Aeon

Bottle #15 Clear/Violet

Use of #15 should begin at age 7, and continue to the onset of Puberty. It will support the child to balance their male and female personality traits, discern and stand in their own truth, and move graciously and without fear into new or expanded social groups or situations.

In addition to these five bottles, one other might be useful to have for after the birth, or if during pregnancy the unborn child starts to fret.

Childs Rescue

Bottle #20 Blue/Pink

#20 is recommended for acute or crisis situations in a child's life, regardless of which stage the child is in. #20 may also be used to combat overly aggressive behaviour in young boys, or conversely support shy or withdrawn female children to be more open, confident and courageous

There are many books dedicated solely to aura soma, and I would recommend reading one of them, I have several bottles in which I use to give a certain aura or feeling to certain rooms, for example, I do most of my magical work in my dining room, rituals, readings etc. therefore I spay the royal blue pomander here to promote a psychic sense, and in the children's bedrooms, I spray El Morya to give a secure loving feeling. The different scents of the bottles are amazing, and the look of the equilibrium bottles is so charming.

The Aura

The aura is made up of seven main auras' which extend up to four feet from the body. These auras's all occupy the same space at the same time, each aura extending out further than the previous aura. All auras are interconnected and reliant on the others for normal function. There are also three higher aura's which I've included.

Auric Levels

Etheric Body

This aura extends about two inches out from the physical body and is usually a shade of blue in colour. The shade of the blue relates to the physical condition and health of the physical body. Athletes have strong etheric auras of a deeper blue in shade. In the etheric aura you feel all the sensations, both pain and pleasure. Whenever there is pain the flow of energy in that area of the etheric is erratic.

Emotional Body

This aura extends about two to four inches from the physical body and appears as rainbow coloured clouds. This aura is associated with feelings. Positive feelings generally create bright colours, where as negative feelings generally create dark colours. Problems in this aura will eventually lead to problems in the first and third auras. This is the one we'll be trying to see afterwards.

Mental Body

This aura extends about four to eight inches from the physical body and is usually a bright shade of yellow in colour. Within this aura are our thoughts and mental processes. The more active our thinking processes the brighter our mental aura becomes. Within this aura can be found thought forms.

Astral Body

The astral aura extends about eight to twelve inches from the physical body and appears as beautifully coloured rainbow clouds. The astral aura is the bridge or link between the physical world and the spiritual world.

Etheric Template Body

The etheric template aura extends about twelve to twenty four inches from the physical body and appears in a kind of blue print form. It is said that there is an empty groove in the etheric aura into which the etheric template aura fits. The etheric template aura holds the etheric aura in place. It is the template for the etheric dimension. Doesn't that sound confusing?

Celestial Body

The celestial aura extends about twenty four inches from the physical body and appears as a brighter shimmering light of pastel colours. This is the level of feelings within the world of our spirit. Here we communicate with all the beings of the spiritual world. Unconsciously of course.

Ketheric or Causal Body

The ketheric template aura extends about thirty six to forty eight inches from the physical body and appears as an extremely bright golden light that is rapidly pulsating. This aura takes on the form of a golden egg that surrounds and protects everything within it. It is like a shield that protects us.

Memory Body

The eighth layer is located at the crown of the head and extends upward between one and three feet above the physical body. It is the Time Layer associated with interfaces from past Akashic Records, present and future karmic memories, or existences.

Soul Body

This auric layer is very small and occupies an almost non-existent space on the physical plane. It is located several inches above the head. The ninth layer is the Soul Body or Soul Level, associated with the planes between the worlds of heaven and now. This layer interfaces with our "oneness" with Deity or Divine in our pre-destined soul contracts. This body is also sometimes known as the Soul Star.

Integrative Body

The tenth layer is located between the physical body and the etheric body. It serves as a pathway between the physical and the spiritual worlds. This is the body which is used during astral projection. It can access data from our genetic and soul heritage and contains imprints of our soul purpose. It is also recognized as the layer which integrates our chakras and spiritual energy centres.

How to See the Aura

Everybody has the ability to see the aura. For beginners a low light is the best way to start.

Turn out the lights and lay on the bed. Leave the window curtains open and let the natural light flow in. As you are lying on the bed hold your hands out at full distance in front of you. Don't stare hard but rather just gaze at your hands. Moving your hands slowly, bring your fingertips together until they are almost touching. You will notice a cloudy blue haze appear around your finger. This is the etheric aura. You could also ask somebody to sit in front of a white wall. Gaze at the person until you see a haze around their shoulders. Just don't leave them sitting there too long!

Feeling the Aura

I personally feel it is far easier to feel the aura, than to see it. Try this small experiment! Draw a circle on your left hand using your right fingertip. Don't let your finger touch your hand, keep it at a distance of about a half inch. Move slowly. You will feel your aura.

The aura of pregnant women and babies

The aura of a pregnant woman is one of the easiest to see, for it is especially bright and full of gold. This explains why a pregnant woman often arouses a feeling of respect, if not awe. Even though the people around her may not be able to see her aura consciously, they unconsciously register some of the golden energy and are impressed by it. And everyone knows that pregnant women glow radiantly.

The gold colour in the aura indicates that the pregnant woman is closely connected to high spiritual beings who support and protect the growing embryo. Pregnancy is therefore a privileged time for spiritual growth. As said before, it's a time to meditate. It can also be used to work at developing intuition and perception. Apart from the fact that the baby is extremely sensitive to the mother's thoughts and emotions and influenced by them, a spiritual focus during pregnancy can bring about positive changes in the mother.

The aura of a new-born baby

The aura of a new born baby is a wonder in itself. It is a bright and luminous light, and relatively easy to see. This may be because, the baby keeps some of the light of the angels that have assisted in the process of birth for a while after birth. The strong participation of the angels in all that is related to birth makes a delivery a most fascinating experience of consciousness. I have yet to hear of a father who does not shed a tear at witnessing the birth of his child.

Apart from the touch of the angels, during its first few days back on Earth the baby is still "wearing" some astral impressions obtained from the journey it has just completed through intermediary worlds. To the lucky empathy or practiced clairvoyant these may be perceived as images that flow into your consciousness as soon as you tune into the child's aura. But it normally needs a very practiced auric reader to see these impressions.

The Sixth Month

This month continues to be a period of rapid growth. Your baby's skin is wrinkled and red. It is covered with lanugo (fine, soft hair) and vernix (a substance consisting of oil, sloughed skin cells and lanugo). Real hair and toenails are beginning to grow. Your baby's brain is developing rapidly. Fatty sheaths which transmit electrical impulses along nerves are forming. Meconium, your baby's first poop (stool), is developing. A special type of fat (brown fat) that keeps your baby warm at birth is forming. Baby girls will develop eggs in their ovaries during this month. The baby's bones are becoming solid.

Your baby is almost fully formed and looks like a tiny human. However, because the lungs are not well developed and the baby is still very small, a baby at this stage normally can't live outside the uterus without highly specialized care.

By the end of the sixth month, Your baby will be around 11 to 14 inches long and will weigh about 1 to 1 1/2 pounds.

What is Happening with You

Continue to see your doctor for all of your prenatal care appointments. It is important that your weight, blood pressure, urine, foetal heartbeat, fundal height, uterus size, swelling, varicose veins, and other symptoms are continually monitored throughout your pregnancy, this is normally the month where I start getting one kidney infection after the other, due to the fact that I have a wandering kidney and it seems to get jammed as the baby grows, thank Deity for Cantharis! (homeopathy).

You will be feeling a lot more foetal activity as your baby grows larger and stronger, his or her bones become solid, and he or she becomes more active. You are likely to still experience lower abdominal aches; leucorrhoea; constipation; heartburn, indigestion, flatulence, or bloating; occasional headaches, faintness, or dizziness; nasal congestion; nosebleeds; ear stuffiness; bleeding gums; a hearty appetite; leg cramps; swelling; backache; varicose veins; enlarged breasts; and skin pigmentation changes. You may also begin to have an itchy abdomen. But who cares, you look great!

Emotionally, absentmindedness, boredom, and anxiety are common during this period of your pregnancy.

What is Happening with Your Partner

Your partner is also probably anxious. Share your feelings about becoming a parent and how it will affect your life. Attend childbirth and parenting classes together to get ready for your new baby. Allow your partner to feel the baby moving and kicking inside of you, but don't force him. Even his blowing of raspberries on your bump, can be a very intimate time for both of you!

Homeopathy

Homeopathy is ideal for treating the niggles of pregnancy, as it carries no side effects

During pregnancy, any conventional medication feels like a threat to the unborn. However, the gentle and ancient system of homeopathy suits pregnancy because it does not introduce harmful substances into the body. With homeopathy, you're not just treating a symptom - nausea, constipation or itchiness, for instance - you're treating the whole pregnant person.

If you go to a Homeopath, remedies are chosen after a consultation, which can include bewildering questions about whether you have hot feet and what you like best to eat. This is in order to establish a complete picture of the patient, to which the homeopath can match a correct remedy. The same symptoms can be treated with a wide variety of different remedies, depending on the person's unique susceptibility. Once the remedy has been identified, it works by stimulating the recipient's healing potential and restoring equilibrium.

Sometimes the effects can seem immediate and startling. For example, high potency Pulsatilla, used towards the end of pregnancy, is recommended for turning a breech baby head downwards. This has been documented many times. So, if your baby is breech and won't turn it's worth consulting a homeopath - it certainly can't do any harm.

Panic stations!

The overwhelming sensations of a first labour can induce panic. If your still in the planning phase of your pregnancy, you might consider consulting a professional homoeopath for care during pregnancy, birth and the post-partum period – (obviously in addition to the medical team at the hospital, or a midwife!) my midwife had extremely good knowledge of homeopathy (among other alternative remedies). There are 'first-aid' remedies that can help with minor or uncomplicated problems, for example Gossypium (cotton) could be used if contractions are irratic and fail to establish properly, I've even heard of it been given to a woman who is gone over her due date. A remedy should be chosen that best matches the general state - as well as the symptoms - of the person.

The digestive system is often affected by pregnancy. Constipation is quite common and is sometimes resolved by a glass of hot water first thing in the morning, and by increasing fibre in the diet. If nausea (whether in the morning or any other time) is a problem, some people find it settles if they eat little and often, especially carbohydrate foods. Ginger in some form (such as ginger beer, fresh ginger tea or ginger biscuits) can also be helpful, but always be careful with ginger.

Finding relief

If symptoms are more persistent, you can try the following remedies:

Sepia - nausea is intensified by the smell of food, yet relieved by eating. Tendency to feel worn out, irritable and over-burdened by her responsibilities, with no spare emotional energy for loved ones. Constipation with sluggish feeling and sense that some stool remains behind.

Pulastilla - nausea with some relief from fresh air. Intolerance of fatty foods and probably not very thirsty. Changeable moods, sometimes weepy. Feels generally better for company, sympathy and possibly cuddles.

Nux Vomica - nausea relieved by vomiting. Indigestion and heartburn; constipation with frequent unproductive urging. Easily irritated, and loss of sleep affects her badly.

Ipecac - continuous nausea that isn't relieved by vomiting. The tongue tends to be a normal pink colour and there may be more saliva than usual.

Bryonia - useful in constipation with large, dry stools. This may be accompanied by a dull headache and dry mouth.

One remedy you will probably be advised to have to help with soreness and bruising after the birth is arnica (to be taken in tablet form as the cream should not be put on broken skin).

Calendula or *hypercal* - (a mixture of calendula and hypericum) tincture mixed with warm water (20 drops in ¼ pint) is very soothing to bathe the perineum after birth, and calendula steam baths are helpful from about the thirtieth week to soften the pelvic floor and perineum and it has been proven that women who use calendula steam baths are less likely to go over their due date.

Caulophyllum - has a great reputation for helping slow labours progress. The characteristic indications are painful yet ineffectual contractions, often with weakness and trembling.

Aconite - is very helpful if a woman in labour feels panicky, if she feels the baby is never going to arrive, and if she can't cope with the labour.

After the baby has arrived, homoeopathic remedies are useful for both mother and infant. Two common problems with breastfeeding are mastitis and thrush. In the beginning stages of mastitis, or threatening breast abscess with pain, heat of the breast and fever, belladonna works in most cases. In thrush, passed to and fro between the baby's mouth and the mother's breasts, borax given to both is often very useful.

Calendula ointment or nappy cream can help heal cracked or sore nipples and also soothe a baby's sore bottom.

How to take remedies

When prescribing for yourself, it is best to try a 6c potency (readily obtained from health food shops and many chemists. If you experience a definite improvement, only repeat the remedy if the improvement starts to wear off.

If there is little or no improvement after one dose, try further doses but no more than six over a couple of days. Avoid coffee, camphor and menthol etc., while taking the remedies. Don't touch them with your fingers (tip from the lid straight under your tongue and let them dissolve slowly). Avoid eating or drinking within half an hour on either side of taking a remedy, which is often difficult when pregnant.

It was at this time that I normally started a Birth list. This is a list where I recorded what I wanted for the birth. For example if you’re going to a hospital, in the heat of the moment , you might not think of telling the staff what you’d like, for example a water birth, aromatherapy scents, homeopathic remedies, epidural, or no medication, limited people coming in and out etc. You could ask your partner to pass this on to the nurse. Why not plan together.

During my third pregnancy, my mood swings were a little too much for me to cope with, so I took pulsatilla in C7, two in the morning and two in the evening for my extreme mood swings until they subsided. And honestly, it's all part of the experience of becoming a mom! Enjoy being able to vent your emotions!!

The Seventh Month

Your baby is continuing to grow and develop. Your baby's eyes can now open and close and can sense light changes. The lanugo is starting to disappear from the baby's face. Your baby's hearing is getting better. He or she can now hear the outside world quite well over the sound of your heartbeat, and may be startled sometimes by a loud noise, but even dad's raspberries will cease to startle after the one hundredth time!. The baby exercises by kicking and stretching. He or she can also make grasping motions and likes to suck its thumb.

By the end of this month, your baby will be approximately 15 inches long and weigh about 2 or 2 1/2 pounds. If the baby was born now, its chances of survival are better than last month.

What is Happening With You

Your doctor will continue to check your weight gain, blood pressure, urine, the fundal height, oedema, varicose veins, and any symptoms you are experiencing. He or she will also check the size and position of the foetus and the foetal heartbeat. If you haven't already, start thinking about any questions you have about labour and delivery and discuss them at your prenatal check-ups.

You are likely to still be experiencing constipation, heartburn, indigestion, flatulence, and bloating. Your lower abdomen may feel achy as well. You may have occasional headaches, faintness, and dizziness. Your leucorrhoea (whitish vaginal discharge) is getting increasingly heavy. Hormonal changes may be causing nasal congestion, occasional nosebleeds, and ear stuffiness. Your gums may still be bleeding and sensitive. Other common physical symptoms include leg cramps, backaches, varicose veins, haemorrhoids, mild swelling, shortness of breath, difficulty sleeping, and clumsiness. You are probably also feeling Braxton Hicks contractions that are usually painless. During a Braxton Hicks contraction, your uterus hardens for a minute and then returns to normal. Colostrum may be leaking from your enlarged breasts.

By this time, women often find themselves feeling bored and a bit weary about their pregnancy. It is normal to feel like you just want this to be over. At the same time, you may also be feeling more and more apprehensive about becoming a mother, your baby's health, and about labour and delivery. Hormonal changes may make you grumpy again and you may be a bit absentminded, or like me, I just couldn't wait to see my baby.

What is Happening with Your Partner

You and your partner are probably both fantasizing and dreaming about your baby and your baby's future. Tell each other your hopes and dreams for your child. You and your partner also should discuss any fears about the increased responsibility involved with becoming a parent. You can work together to prioritize responsibilities and decide how the two of you can share the workload.

Making a mobile

Mobiles were invented by the American sculptor Alexander Calder in the early 20th century, babies are fascinated with them and they are fairly easy to make. You can hang it over baby's bed or changing table. Try sticking to bright colours, as baby notices them more

Using twigs for the "arms" of the mobile, and Fimo or thin wood to make stars, moons, animals or whatever else you may find pretty.

It doesn't have to be complicated, just five pieces of string (one to hang up!), four shapes and two twigs or sticks! Baby will love it, and the designs are limitless!

If you're pagan, why not use the idea of a mobile to create a protection spell, or a health spell! Use protective symbols in bright colours.

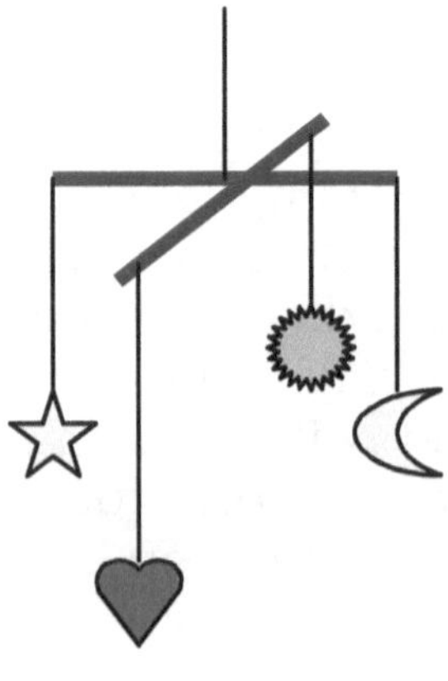

The Eight Month

Your baby's body continues to grow quickly. The bones are getting stronger, limbs are fatter, and the skin has a healthy glow. The brain is now forming its different regions. The brain and nerves are directing bodily functions. Taste buds are developing. Your baby may now hiccup, cry, taste sweet and sour, and respond to pain, light, and sound. If you are having a boy, his testicles have dropped from his abdomen where they will then descend into his scrotum. Almost fully developed!

Your baby will be about 16 to 18 inches long and will weigh about 4 pounds at the end of this month.

What is Happening with You

After your 32nd week, your doctor will probably want you to come in more often, about every two weeks so that your pregnancy can be more closely monitored. He or she will assess the health of you and your baby by checking your weight, blood pressure, urine, foetal heartbeat, fundal height, size and position of the foetus, oedema, varicose veins, and other symptoms. Discuss your birthing plan with your provider and pain management during labour and delivery. Come to your appointments prepared with a list of questions and problems you want to discuss.

You will be feeling strong, regular foetal activity, kicks in the ribs and jabs to the stomach!. Your baby's kicks are strong and you may even be able to see the outline of a small heel or elbow against your abdomen, that is if you can tell which it is!. Many of the discomforts you have been experiencing the last few months with constipation and shortness of breath are becoming more of a problem. Braxton Hicks contractions will increase. Your navel will begin to stick out if it doesn't already.

Eagerness to have the pregnancy over and apprehension about the baby's health and labour and delivery are probably increasing. You will also be more clumsy and absentminded, your centre of gravity has shifted a lot, so clumsiness is probably an understatement! You don't have much longer to wait! And believe me, you're going to miss all these symptoms, even the less pleasant ones!

What is Happening With Your Partner

Couvade, the occurrence of pregnancy-like symptoms in expecting fathers, may return in your partner. He may be feeling depressed and tired and may gain weight. Increased communication can help him with these feelings. Attend childbirth preparation classes together. It's a long nine months for him too!

While it is important for you and your partner to be discussing your baby and the plans for your growing family, it is also a good idea to take a break from all of this childbirth and baby planning so that you and your partner can experience some romance again. Once a week, try to make a date to do something together that is fun, romantic, and has nothing to do with babies. Taking a break for romance won't make the wonderful event any less special but it will do wonders for the relationship between the two of you. It doesn’t have to be much, even a walk to the park to feed the ducks can be romantic. (That is if the ducks don’t remind you or him of your clumsiness. You could end up I a fit of laughter!)

Boar's Teeth

The following is taken from Charles Godfrey Leland's book, Gypsy Sorcery and Fortune Telling, published in 1891, it is an excellent book to read. I love reading old literature, the older the better. There is a lot of lost information in old books and one can get a good picture of how people thought in the past.

Leland writes that the boar's tooth, has been a charm since time immemorial; He found them attached to chatelaines and bunches of keys, especially in Austria, from one to four or five centuries past. They were also found in prehistoric graves. The tusk is probably a male emblem; a pig is sometimes placed on the base. These were still very commonly made and sold in Leland's time. He saw one worn by the son of a travelling basket-maker, who spoke Romany, and personally purchased several in Vienna in 1888, and in Copenhagen in 1889. In Florence very large boars' tusks were set as brooches, and could be found generally in the smaller jewellers' shops and on the Ponte Vecchio. They were regarded as protective against malocchio, a general term for evil influences or the evil eye, especially for women during pregnancy, and as securing plenty, i.e., prosperity and increase, be it of worldly goods, honour, or prosperity. He also tells of a boar's tusk, mounted or set as an amulet, in the museum in Budapest which was apparently of Celtic origin, and which certainly belonged to the migration of races, or a very early period. And it was in this eastern portion of Europe that it was most widely used or worn as a charm.

I thought it would be interesting to mention that little piece of information about the charm here, many people nowadays still wear certain types of jewellery to protect their baby during pregnancy. From holy saint's medals, to copies of ancients charms and ornaments. If you are so inclined, you could do some research on the typical types of jewellery or charms customary in your country.

The ninth Month

Yippee almost there! Your baby is now gaining about a 1/2 pound each week. Your baby is getting plumper and its skin is less rumpled. He or she is getting ready for birth and is settling into the foetal position with its head down against the birth canal, its legs tucked up to its chest, and its knees against its nose.

Your antibodies to disease are beginning to flow rapidly through the placenta. The rapid flow of blood through the umbilical cord keeps it taut which prevents tangles.

Your baby is beginning to develop sleeping patterns. Your baby will continue to kick and punch although it will move lower in your abdomen to under your pelvis (this is a process called "lightening"). You will also feel your baby roll around as it gets too cramped inside your uterus for much movement. Your baby's lungs are now mature and your baby will have a great chance of survival if born a little early. The bones of baby's head are soft and flexible to ease the process of delivery through the birth canal.

Your baby is now about 20 inches long and weighs approximately 6 to 9 pounds. Your baby may be born anytime between the 37th and 42nd week of pregnancy. Only 5 percent of babies are born on their due date.

What is Happening with You

After your 36th week, your doctor will increase your prenatal appointments to weekly. Your provider will check your weight, blood pressure, urine, fundal height, oedema, and varicose veins. He or she will also check the foetal heartbeat, size, presentation (head or buttocks first?), position (facing the front or the back?), and descent. Your cervix will be examined sometime after the 38th week for effacement and dilation (opening of the cervix). You will ask to report on the frequency and duration of your Braxton Hicks contractions. Ask any questions you have, especially about labour and delivery. You should also receive instructions as when to call if you think you are in labour. If you do not receive these instructions, ask for them.

You will feel changes in the foetal activity (more squirming and rolling and less kicking). Leucorrhoea will become heavier and will contain more mucus. It may be streaked with blood or tinged brown or pink after intercourse or pelvic exam. In addition to the pregnancy discomforts you have been feeling the last couple of months, you may have some discomfort and achiness in your buttocks and pelvic area, increased backache and heaviness, more difficulty sleeping, and more frequent and intense Braxton Hicks contractions (which may now be painful). Due to the lower position of your baby, it will be easier for you to breathe but you will need to urinate more frequently. You may feel very fatigued or have extra energy or alternate between the two. Your appetite may be increased or diminished substantially.

You will likely be feeling more excited, anxious, apprehensive, and relieved that it is almost over. You may feel irritable, overly sensitive, restless, and impatient. All of these feelings are normal. Don't worry--you won't be pregnant much longer!

Remember to pack your bag so that you will be ready to rush to the hospital when the time comes.

What is Happening with Your Partner

Your partner is likely to be feeling much the same "mixed bag" of emotions as you are as well as being concerned with your health and comfort during labour and delivery. Continue communicating with each other about your feelings. Have your partner pack clothes for sleeping at the hospital so he or she will be ready when it is finally time to deliver your baby.

Packing for the Hospital or Birth House

What to pack in your Birth bag!

- Lip Balm
- Watch with second hand
- Tooth brushes and Tooth paste
- Any reference book or pamphlet you might need
- Music you would like (You may need to provide your own CD Player or Tape Player)
- Camera with film and batteries
- Camcorder with charged batteries and accessories
- Signed copies of your birth plan
- Waterproof pads for the car ride
- Any clothes of your own that you wish to wear
- List of people to call after the baby is born
- Massage items (Oils, massagers, etc.)
- Change of clothes for partner, including swim trunks for shower
- Baby Book for getting the foot prints done by the nurse when she does the paperwork

- Focal Point (If you want one)
- Socks for mom
- Special foods or drinks
- Snacks for labour support
- Calling Card for Long Distance Calls
- Anything else you think you can use (Candles, pictures, etc.)

Your Postpartum Bag

- Nursing bras
- Going home outfit for baby
- More film

- Another change of clothes for partner
- Your own personal night gown robe (They will get dirty!)
- Personal Hygiene items (shampoo, your own sanitary pads, etc.)
- Number of diaper service (if you need to arrange for delivery)
- Car Seat
- Blanket for Baby
- Going home outfit for mom (You will still look about 6 months pregnant)
- Birth Announcements

Premature Labor

What is premature labour?

Premature or pre-term labour is labour that begins more than three weeks before you are expected to deliver your baby, after the thirty-seventh week your baby is mature, or ready to be born. Contractions cause the cervix to open earlier than normal.

Pre-term labour may result in the birth of a premature baby, one of the biggest problems facing premature infants is underdeveloped lungs. However, labour often can be stopped to allow the baby more time to grow and develop in the uterus. Treatments to stop premature labour may include bed rest, fluids given intravenously, and medications to relax the uterus.

There are times when premature labour should not be stopped; for instance, if there is an infection or if the foetus is in distress. If born prematurely after the seventh month, a baby would likely survive, but may need to stay for a short time in the neonatal intensive care unit (NICU) of the hospital. If the baby is born earlier than the seventh month, he or she may be able to survive with specialized care in the NICU.

What are the signs of premature labour?

It is important for you to learn the signs of premature labour so that you can recognize them and get help to stop it and prevent your baby from being born too early. Premature labour is usually not painful, but there are several warning signs, including:

- Four or more contractions or tightening of the muscles in the uterus in one hour, it is difficult to tell the difference between these and brackton hicks contractions, and only a doctor will know

- Regular tightening or low, dull pain in your back that either comes or goes or is constant (but is not relieved by changing positions or other comfort measures)

- Lower abdominal cramping that may feel like gas pain (with or without diarrhoea)

- Increased pressure in the pelvis or vagina

- Menstrual-like cramps

- Increased vaginal discharge, or bloody discharge

- Leaking of fluid from the vagina Vaginal bleeding

- Decreased foetal movements (the baby does not kick as often as it usually does)

What should I do if I have signs of premature labour?

Call your health care provider right away if you have:

- Leaking of fluid from the vagina
- Vaginal bleeding
- Sudden increase of vaginal discharge

Lie down and check for contractions if you have any of the following signs of premature labour:

- Menstrual-like cramps or abdominal cramps
- Low, dull backache
- Pelvic or vaginal pressure
- Vaginal discharge changes

To check for contractions, place your fingertips on your abdomen. If you can feel your uterus tightening and softening, you can then record how often the contractions are happening. To time your contractions, at the beginning of one contraction and again at the beginning of the next contraction, write down the time.

If you have four or more contractions in one hour that do not go away after changing your position or relaxing, call your health care provider. Also call your health care provider if the warning signs listed above do not go away in one hour or if pain is severe and persistent.

What happens if I have to go to the hospital?
After talking to your health care provider about your signs of premature labour, he or she may tell you to go to the hospital. Once you arrive:

- You will be asked to wear a hospital gown.
- You will be given fluids.
- Your pulse, blood pressure and temperature will be checked.
- A monitor will be placed on your abdomen to check the baby's heart rate and evaluate uterine contractions, this will normally be monitored for about a half hour to an hour.
- Your cervix will be checked to see if it is opening.

If you are in premature labour, you may receive medication to stop labour so your baby has more time to develop in the uterus, sometimes a steroid injection will be given to speed up the maturing of the lungs. If the labour has progressed and cannot be stopped, you may need to deliver your baby. If you are not in premature labour, you will be able to go home.

The Celtic Tree Horoscope

I love horoscopes, and it was always a topic greatly discussed during my pregnancies.... what star sign will the baby be born under? Well we all know about the "normal" horoscope signs, and even the Chinese horoscope is reliving a great come back the past few years. But one of my favourites would have to be the Celtic tree horoscope. Being Irish, I guess it's just in my blood. Well here's the list of Celtic tree signs for you to look through, I hope you have as much fun as I always had pondering the future sign and character of my unborn baby.

Birch - The Achiever

December 24 – January 20

If you were born under the energy of the Birch you can be highly driven, and often motivate others they become easily caught in your zeal, drive and ambition. You are always reaching for more, seeking better horizons and obtaining higher aspirations. The Druids attributed this to your time of birth, which is a time of year shrouded by darkness, so consequently you are always stretching out to find the light. Birch signs (just like the tree) are tolerant, tough, and resilient. You are cool-headed and are natural-born rulers, often taking command when a situation calls for leadership. When in touch with your softer side, you also bring beauty in otherwise barren spaces, brightening up a room with you guile, and charming crowds with you quick wit. Celtic tree astrology Birch signs are compatible with Vine signs and Willow signs.

Rowan - The Thinker

January 21 – February 17

Celtic tree astrology recognizes Rowan signs as the philosophical minds within the zodiac. If you were born under the Rowan energy, you are likely a keen-minded visionary, with high ideals. Your thoughts are original and creative, so much so, that other's often misunderstand from where you are coming. This sometimes makes you aloof when interacting with others as you feel they wouldn't understand where you are coming from anyway.

Nevertheless, although you may appear to have a cool exterior, you are burning within from your passionate ideals. This inner passion provides inner motivation for you as you make your way through life. You have a natural ability to transform situations and people around you by your mere presence. You are highly influential in a quiet way and others look to you for your unique perspectives. Rowan pairs well with Ivy and Hawthorn signs.

Ash - The Enchanter

February 18 – March 17

Those born under the Celtic tree astrology sign of the Ash are free thinkers. Imaginative, intuitive, and naturally artistic, you see the world in water-colour purity. You have a tendency to moody and withdrawn at times, but that's only because your inner landscape is in constant motion. You are in touch with your muse, and you are easily inspired by nature. Likewise, you inspire all that you associate with and people seek you out for your enchanting personality. Art, writing (especially poetry), science, and theology (spiritual matters) are areas that strongly interest you. Others may think you are reclusive, but in all honesty, you are simply immersed in your own world of fantastic vision and design. You are in a constant state of self-renewal and you rarely place a value on what others think about you. Ash signs partner well with Willow and Reed signs

Alder - The Trailblazer

March 18 – April 14

If you are an Alder sign within the Celtic tree astrology system, you are a natural-born pathfinder. You're a mover and a shaker, and will blaze a trail with fiery passion often gaining loyal followers to your cause. You are charming, gregarious and mingle easily with a broad mix of personalities. In other words, Alder signs get along with everybody and everybody loves to hang around with you. This might be because Alder's are easily confident and have a strong self-faith. This self-assurances is infectious and other people recognize this quality in you instantly. Alder Celtic tree astrology signs are very focused and dislike waste. Consequently, they can see through superficialities and will not tolerate fluff. Alder people place high value on their time, and feel that wasting time is insufferable. They are motivated by action and results. Alder's pair well with Hawthorns, Oaks or even Birch signs

Willow - The Observer

April 15 – May 12

If you are a Willow sign, you are ruled by the moon, and so your personality holds hands with many of the mystical aspects of the lunar realm. This means you are highly creative, intuitive (highly psychic people are born under the sign of the Willow) and intelligent. You have a keen understanding of cycles, and you inherently know that every situation has a season. This gives you a realistic perspective of things, and also causes you to be more patient than most tree signs. With your intelligence comes a natural ability to retain knowledge and you often impress your company with the ability to expound on subjects from memory. Willow Celtic tree astrology signs are bursting with potential, but have a tendency to hold themselves back for fear of appearing flamboyant or overindulgent. It is your powers of perception that ultimately allow your true nature to shine, and what leads you to success in life. Willow signs join well with the Birch and the Ivy.

Hawthorn - The Illusionist

May 13 – June 9

Hawthorn signs in Celtic tree astrology are not at all what they appear to be. Outwardly, they appear to be a certain persona, while on the inside Hawthorn's are quite different. They put the term "never judge a book by its cover" to the test. They live seemingly average lives while on the inside they carry fiery passions and inexhaustible creative flame. They are well adjusted and can adapt to most life situations well – making themselves content and comforting others at the same time. You are naturally curious, and have an interest in a broad range of topics. You are an excellent listener, and people seek you out as an outlet to release their burdens. You have a healthy sense of humour, and have a clear understanding of irony. You tend to see the big picture, and have amazing insight – although you typically won't give yourself enough credit for your observations. Hawthorn signs match up nicely with Ash and Rowan's.

Oak - The Stabilizer

June 10 – July 7

Those born under the Celtic tree astrology sign of the Oak have a special gift of strength. They are protective people and often become a champion for those who do not have a voice. In other words, the Oak is the crusader and the spokesperson for the underdog. Nurturing, generous and helpful, you are a gentle giant among the Celtic zodiac signs. You exude an easy confidence and naturally assume everything will work out to a positive outcome. You have a deep respect for history and ancestry, and many people with this sign become teachers. You love to impart your knowledge of the past to others. Oak signs have a need for structure, and will often go to great lengths to gain the feeling of control in their lives. Healthy Oak signs live long, full, happy lives and enjoy large family settings and are likely to be involved with large social/community networks. Oak signs pair off well with the Ash and Reed, and are known to harmoniously join with Ivy signs too.

Holly - The Ruler

July 8 – August 4

Among the Celtic tree astrology signs the Holly is one of regal status. Noble, and high-minded, those born during the Holly era easily take on positions of leadership and power. If you are a Holly sign you take on challenges easily, and you overcome obstacles with rare skill and tact. When you encounter setbacks, you simply redouble your efforts and remain ever vigilant to obtain your end goals. Very seldom are you defeated. This is why many people look up to you and follow you as their leader. You are competitive and ambitious even in the most casual settings. You can appear to be arrogant but in actuality you're just very confident in your abilities. Truth be known, you are quite generous, kind and affectionate (once people get to know you). Highly intelligent, you skate through academics where others may struggle. Because many things come to you so easily, you may have a tendency to rest on your laurels. In other words, if not kept active, you may slip into an unhealthy and lazy lifestyle. Holly signs may look to Ash and Elder signs for balance and partnership.

Hazel - The Knower

August 5 – September 1

If you are born under the energy of the Hazel, you are highly intelligent, organized and efficient. Like the Holly, you are naturally gifted in academia, and excel in the classroom. You also have the ability to retain information and can recall, recite and expound on subjects you've memorized with amazing accuracy. You know your facts, and you are always well informed. This sometimes makes you appear like a know-it-all to others, but you can't help that; you're genuinely smart and usually know the right course of action because of your impressive knowledge base. You have an eye for detail, and like things to be "just so." Sometimes this need for order and control can lead to compulsive behaviours if left unchecked. You have a knack for numbers, science and things that utilize your analytical skills. You like rules, although you are typically making them rather than playing by them. The Celtic tree astrology sign of Hazel joins harmoniously with Hawthorn and Rowan's.

Vine - The Equalizer

September 2 – September 29

Vine signs are born within the autumnal equinox, which makes your personality changeable and unpredictable. You can be full of contradictions, and are often indecisive. But this is because you can see both sides of the story, and empathize with each equally. It is hard for you to pick sides because you can see the good points on each end. There are, however, areas in your life that you are quite sure about. These include the finer things of life like food, wine, music, and art. You have very distinctive taste, and are a connoisseur of refinement. Luxury agrees with you, and under good conditions you have a Midas touch for turning drab into dramatic beauty. You are charming, elegant, and maintain a level of class that wins you esteem from a large fan base. Indeed, you often find yourself in public places where others can admire your classic style and poise. Vine signs pair well with Willow and Hazel signs.

Ivy - The Survivor

September 30 – October 27

Among other cherished qualities of the Ivy Celtic tree astrology sign, most prized is your ability to overcome all odds. You have a sharp intellect, but more obvious is your compassion and loyalty to others. You have a giving nature, and are always there to lend a helping hand. You are born at a time of the waning sun so life can be difficult for you at times. This sometimes seems unfair because it appears that obstacles are coming at with no prompting on your part. Nevertheless, you endure troubling times with silent perseverance and soulful grace. Indeed, Ivy signs have a tendency to be deeply spiritual and cling to a deep-rooted faith that typically sees them through adversity. You are soft spoken, but have a keen wit about you. You are charming, charismatic, and can effectively hold your own in most social settings. Ivy signs are attracted to the Celtic tree astrology sign of Oak and Ash signs.

Reed - The Inquisitor

October 28 – November 24

Reed signs among the Celtic tree astrology signs are the secret keepers. You dig deep inside to the real meaning of things and discover the truth hidden beneath layers of distraction. When there is a need to get to the heart of the matter, most certainly the Reed sign will find the core. You love a good story, and can be easily drawn in by gossip, scandals, legend and lore. These tendencies also make you an excellent historian, journalist, detective or archaeologist. You love people because they represent a diversity of meanings for you to interpret. You are adept at coaxing people to talking to you, and sometimes you can be a bit manipulative. However, you have a strong sense of truth and honour so most of your scheming is harmless. Reed people join well with other Reeds, Ash or Oak signs.

Elder - The Seeker

November 25 – December 23

Elder archetypes among Celtic tree astrology tend to be freedom-loving, and sometimes appear to be a bit wild to the other signs of the zodiac. In younger years you may have lived life in the fast lane, often identified as a "thrill seeker." At the time of your birth the light of the sun was fast fleeting and so you take the same cue from nature. You are often misjudged as an outsider as you have a tendency to be withdrawn in spite of your extroverted nature. In actuality, you are deeply thoughtful with philosophical bent. You also tend to be very considerate of others and genuinely strive to be helpful. These acts of assistance are sometimes thwarted by your brutal honestly (which you openly share solicited or otherwise). Elder Celtic tree astrology signs fit well with Alder's and Holly's.

Divers Trivia!

Salomons Shield

This amulet comes from the book of Raziel, that is currently held in the British museum. It is said to be very protective against all negative influences. And it is reputed to be an excellent amulet for pregnant women and new born babies.

In Ireland just about every baby you see has a small either pink or blue plaque pinned to their pram, cot, basket and just about everywhere, where baby lies around. These are small prayer or blessing plaques with a small miraculous medal.

The medal is the one given to Bernadette in Lourdes, and the prayer is as follows;

Watch over him (her) lord
This child that we love
Watch over him (her) lord
From your heaven above
Keep him (her) from harm
Loved let him (her) be
Watch over him (her) lord
As you watched over me

In Switzerland, almost every child from birth up to about seven or eight years old has an amber bead necklace. It is said that these necklaces help teething children, and ease other pains and aches. Not to mention it makes them beautiful too.

The following is a little poem that almost everybody knows, it's a child's rhyme about the day you were born.

Monday's child is fair of face!
Tuesday's child is full of grace
Wednesday's child is full of woe
Thursday's child has far to go
Friday's child is loving and giving
Saturday's child works hard for a living

And the child that is born on the Sabbath day, is
bonny and bright, good and Gay!

Patron Saints

As you most probably know, there is a patron Saint for just about every cause or condition. Here are a couple associated with pregnancy and childbirth.

Pregnant Women - St. Gerard, St. Raymond

Midwives - St. Raymond

Infertility - Saint Anthony

Childbirth - St. Anne, St. Gerard, St. Ramon

Birth Prep

The best way to get ready for the birth is to learn what is going to happen so that you won't be surprised or unready. Knowing what's happening also reduces the need for pain killers and the risk of fretting!

Pre-Labour:

Signs that Labour is About to Begin

Possible Signs

Labour May Begin Soon.

- Backache: Not the type of backache you have in late pregnancy that changes when you shift position, but a persistent dull ache that makes you restless and irritable.
- Cramps. Abdominal cramping that is mild to moderate in discomfort.
- PMS symptoms: crabby, irritable.
- Nesting Urge.
- Frequent, soft bowel movements. Flu-like symptoms.

If you experience any of these symptoms, remember that they are not necessarily signs that labour is imminent. They may a few days or weeks before labour begins, or a few hours. The presence of these symptoms is a good reminder to make sure you have everything prepared for labour and birth, and to make sure you are aware of what other signs to be watching for.

However, try not to get too excited about things, or start calling your partner home from work assuming the baby is on its way. Continue your normal routines, get lots of rest, eat and drink well, nurture yourself in these precious days or hours before the baby arrives.

Preliminary Signs

The following are signs that labour is about to begin, although it could be still 24 hours away, so don't call your partner yet! But be ready just the same.

- Bloody show. During pregnancy, the cervix contains mucus, which may be released in late pregnancy. This may be a thick 'plug' of pinkish mucus, which might come out when you use the toilet. Or it may be a thin, mucousy discharge on toilet paper. If there is more blood than mucus, call your doctor or midwife. (Note, it's common to have a brownish, bloody discharge within 24 hours of a vaginal exam, or intercourse. Don't mistake this for bloody show.)
- Water breaks: Trickle or a gush. If it's just a little mucousy fluid, it may be the mucous

plug. Pay attention to what time it breaks, note down its colour, odour, etc. Call your doctor or midwife. Usually (80% of the time), you will go into labour on your own in the next 24 hours. Ask your caregiver what will happen if you are not in labour after 24 hours.

- Contractions. What's the difference between non-progressing Braxton-Hicks contractions ("false labour" / pre-labour) and the progressive contractions of active labour? Pre-labour contractions are generally irregular, or may stay same length, strength, and frequency. They normally last only for a short time, subsiding after you lie down.. Discomfort is mostly felt in the front of the abdomen, as muscles tighten up. Contractions may stop if you walk, change position or change activity, eat, drink, or empty bladder.

Some women never have Braxton-Hicks, and other may have them for weeks before labour starts. Some may even have several episodes where contractions seem to be developing a pattern: with contractions every 6-7 minutes for 2-3 hours, which then stop again.

'False Labour' doesn't mean they don't hurt, and it also doesn't mean that they're not doing anything. Although the contractions might not be dilating your cervix yet, they are helping you to progress in other ways: moving the cervix to an anterior position, ripening and effacing it.

Positive Signs of Labour

Now we're getting to the call your partner type signs!

- Gush of amniotic fluid from vagina.
- Progressing contractions: Get longer, stronger, and/or closer together with time. Are usually described as 'very strong' or "painful', felt in the abdomen, back, or both. May start in the back, and radiate around to front. Usually increase if you walk. I always had pain in my hips or the top outer sides of my legs.
- Dilation of cervix seen in vaginal exam if you're allowing your midwife to do them.

What's happening: Cervix effaces 50-100%, dilates to 4 cm. Contractions 7-30 minutes apart, 15-45 seconds long. You can walk and talk during contractions.

Your response to your first contractions shouldn't be to pack your bag and rush to the hospital. That's only what happens in the movies, I wasn't actually sure if it was contractions or not, I waited for an hour, all the time watching the clock.

This is early labour. It can last from 2 – 24 hours or more, some women don't even notice it happening! Midwives often say "give it a day." For most pregnancies, it's best to remain home for early labour, and you'll probably be more comfortable at home anyway. Try to keep yourself relaxed, and your labour will progress on its own without you worrying about every contraction. If you're comfortable with the contractions without using special "comfort techniques", that's fine. Don't work harder than you have to!

Comfort in Early Labour.

Ideas for taking care of yourself and helping labour move along, most probably you just need a distraction so it won't seen to pass so slowly

Relaxed Abdominal Breathing, start and end each contraction with a deep cleansing breath.

- Distractions: Go to work. Go shopping, bake a cake, hang out with friends, play cards, work on a hobby. These all help you from getting too obsessed with your contractions too soon. Don't worry, when your contractions need your full attention, you'll know!
- Rest. If it's night-time, let your partner sleep! Try to go back to sleep.
- Take a walk.
- Vary positions: standing, sitting, leaning against wall, sitting on birth ball.
- Eat
- Drink whenever thirsty.
- Go to the bathroom at least once an hour.
- Take a shower.
- Relax muscles during contractions. Relax fully in between contractions.

It is easy to get excited as soon as early labour begins, focusing on every contraction, trying out every comfort technique you have learned, and preparing to leave for the hospital. However, if your waters haven't broken yet, it's always best to stay relaxed and at home.

Call your doctor or midwife if you have questions. If he or she says "you could go to the hospital to be checked if you would like to", ask whether he is saying that just to give you something to do, or because he really thinks it's the right time to go to the hospital. If you do go to the hospital too early, you could find yourself going back home frustrated!

Active Labour. (Active Phase of Stage 1)

What's happening: Cervix is completely effaced, goes from 4-8 cm dilation. Contractions are 3-5 minutes apart, lasting 40-70 seconds. Contractions become more painful.

This phase can last anywhere from 30 minutes to 10 hours. The expectation for progress during this time is 1 cm dilation per hour; although you will only know how much your dilating if you're having regular cervical exams. I don't like being touched during this phase!

Mom's Mood. One of the biggest indicators that active labour has begun is a big change in mom's mood: a lot of women suddenly become much more serious. During a contraction, the contraction takes all of your energy and concentration: you probably can't walk and talk during a contraction anymore. Distractions in between contractions; may start to irritate you now!

This can be a good time to go to the hospital. A standard rule is 5-1-1. Contractions are less than 5 minutes apart, 1 minute long, and have followed that pattern for at least an hour. Plus mom's mood has changed, as described above. If they're more than 5 minutes apart, they're generally not changing the cervix much yet. If mom is still chatty between contractions, even in contractions are intense, she's generally not yet in active labour. If this is not your first baby, labour normally goes at a quicker pace to first time moms.

When asked "How do I know I'm in active labour?" people say "Oh, believe me, you'll know!" But I think it's better to say, when you start to feel like you've got a giant rubber band around your underbelly, that someone tightens and let's go every five minutes!

Comfort Techniques for Active Labour

- Warm water: Baths are wonderful. Generally, don't stay in bath for more than 1 ½ hours at a time. Submerse belly, or have support person pour water over your belly during contractions.
- Breathing: I'm not one for panting, I found very long really deep breaths better. I blew out for most of the contraction. Blowing out helps the belly muscles harden, thus helping ease out baby.

On my third baby, I didn't actually push baby out. I breathed him out, and my midwife agreed to let me do this as long as baby didn't show any signs of distress. My midwife later told me it was a really wonderful, magical experience. My baby was born as the sun was beginning to set. There was an orange glow in the room, and even baby made no sound at all.

I guess, practice makes perfect!

- Positions: Walking, sitting on a Birth Ball, "Slow Dancing" with partner rubbing your back, Hands-and-Knees, Sitting up, leaning over, lunge, squatting, supported squat.
- Eat, if desired. Only mild, easily digested foods, like apple sauce. Not fatty or spicy foods, I'm talking from experience here! Many hospitals do not allow you to eat once you arrive there.
- Drink water after every contraction. If liquid makes you nauseous, try ice chips, popsicles. (Note, nausea and vomiting are fairly common during active labour. Vomiting isn't pleasant, but can be part of a normal labour, and generally isn't cause for concern.)
- Go to bathroom at least once an hour. (A full bladder can block baby's descent.)
- Vocalization: Moaning, Chants, Mantra, Songs. If you find yourself making high-pitched cries, try to bring the tone down to deep belly moaning. This helps you breathe from your abdomen, staying more centred, and less anxious.
- Visualization. Especially images like buds opening up into flowers...know your baby is descending.
- Touch: Effleurage, Counter-pressure, Massage.

- Sensory Distraction: Music, Focal Point, Counting, etc.
- Heat and Cold: Heating Pad or cold packs on back or belly. Cold cloth on head
- Positive feedback.
- Ritual is very important: doing the same thing on every contraction can help keep things calm and familiar.

Cervical dilation does not happen in a straight line of progress, with any guarantees like: every hour of labour is guaranteed to give you 1 cm of dilation. During early labour cervical dilation tends to happen very slowly, your body is only warming up. Sometimes women labour for several hours, and finally decide to go to the hospital, to find out they're only 3 cm dilated. But don't fret, your body will pick up speed, it just has to get used to labouring! Underneath you can see Friedman's Labour Curve notice the shape of the curve, this is how dilation will progress, slowly first, picking up speed. But don't take this chart literally! Every labour is different and varies greatly, these are only averages! Some labours may take less time, some perfectly normal labours may take much more time.

Often women 'plateau' for a while: some women will dilate quickly to 4 cm, and then stay at 4 cm for a long time before shifting into active labour. This is normal, and it's important you're your partner to reinforce that this is a reasonable way for labour to progress.

Another common plateau is when the cervix is almost completely dilated, sometimes there will be a "lip" – just a little bit of the cervix left to efface and dilate before pushing begins.

Transition. (End of First Stage)

What's Happening: Cervix dilates fully from 8 to 10 cm. Contractions are only 2-3 minutes apart, and may 60-90 seconds. Physically and emotionally, this stage of labour is *very* intense for mom, and is usually the most difficult part.

Duration: Range: 10 minutes to 2.5 hours. Average is about 1 hour in first time moms.

Mom's mood: Because of the intensity of transition, mom's moods may be volatile. You may be irritable, hostile, confused, disoriented; you may feel trapped and want to go home; may fear you are dying; often very dependent; discouraged or exhausted. It is common for you to say: "I can't, I can't."

Mom's Physical State: Again, because of the physical intensity of labour, mom may shake all over, your limbs may tremble, you might have nausea and vomiting, prickly feeling on your skin, extreme sensitivity to touch, may feel very hot then very cold, may be belching or passing gas, perspiring, or having muscle cramps, but if you know this is normal, and are expecting it, it won't be so frightening! I actually got giddy at this stage, giggling because I was shaking so bad.

What your Partner can do:

- Assistance with comforting specific physical concerns (e.g. warm blankets, cool cloths, massaging a cramp, etc.)

- Be sensitive to cues, and try to follow her lead; her needs may change from moment to moment, so what was working before may no longer work. And if she's snappy with you, tell her you love her!

- Give short, simple directions. Don't ask a lot of questions: if you need to ask something, make the question specific. Offer 2 options to choose from; don't ask "what can I do for you?" This is very important! She's going to be really into things now and the last thing she needs is someone asking silly questions, it makes you seem helpless, and right now she'll probably want someone to lend her strength.

- Don't leave her alone. Stay within arm's reach.

- Keep your face close to hers; with direct eye contact.

- Breathe with her to help her focus on breathing techniques.

- Most important: reassure her. Let her know she's OK, that these are normal signs of transition, and that labour is nearing its end. Be supportive, and stay as calm and grounded yourself as you possibly can.

Take Charge Routine

Sometimes a mom will have a really hard time with transition. Her support person should move in very close and ask her to keep her eyes open so they can establish clear eye contact. He then should speak calmly and authoritatively, giving specific instructions about breathing, to help her focus again.

She may not be able to calm down, relax and focus at this point, so this should not be your goal. Just work to find some effective coping techniques and a ritual for handling the contractions.

Second Stage of Labour: Birthing the Baby yippee!

Now it's going to get a little easier!

Your cervix is completely effaced, and dilated to 10 cm.

Your baby is turning and getting into position to be born. After the head has been born, baby will again rotate so the shoulders will slip out easily.

During labour, the baby descends into the pelvis. The measurement of this is "station."I never heard of this before I gave birth myself, you will hear this term first during the last few weeks of pregnancy, when your belly starts to move down or sink! When the baby is "floating" high above the pelvic inlet, that is station -4 or -5, because he is 4 or 5 cm above the mom's Ischia spine (the bony knobs at the bottom of your pelvis; sometimes you can feel these when sitting on a hard surface.) The baby is defined as 0 station, or **engaged** (now this one you've probably heard before), when his 'presenting part' (usually his head) is even with the Ischia spine. Many women are at 0 station when labour begins. At +2 or +3, his head is at the vaginal opening, and the perineum is bulging. Crowning, when his head is emerging, is considered +4 or +5 station.

Urge to push.

During second stage contractions, the pressure of baby's in the vagina, and the pressure on the rectum, can cause a strongly felt need to grunt or to hold breath, and to bear down. This urge can be as irresistible as the urge to sneeze or the urge to vomit; resisting it can be more difficult than simply surrendering and letting it happen. The urge may come several times during each contraction. Not all women experience the urge to push, even when unmedicated. With epidural, the urge may be minimal or non-existent.

Duration:

Anywhere from 5 minutes to three or more hours is "normal." Textbook average is 1.5 hours for first time moms, and physicians may encourage interventions past this point.

Mom's Mood.

Some women describe pushing as a relief. Others describe second stage as the most difficult and uncomfortable stage of labour. I personally found it less intense than transition. For many, it's a combination of both of these reactions.

Phases of Second Stage.

Latent.

Not everyone experiences the latent stage. For those who do, it's a time when contractions become less frequent, and there's no strong urge to push. Pushing during this phase doesn't accomplish much, it's better to wait until contractions intensify again. Don't try to rush the birth. If latent phase lasts more than 20-30 minutes may want to try more upright positions to encourage the urge to push. I can't remember any latent phase, but that doesn't mean it didn't happen. Maybe it wasn't important enough to register!

Active / Descent.

Contractions are strong and frequent. Irresistible urge to push. May pass stool or gas. Many women become vocal: grunting, growling, yelling. An excuse to yell at your partner for not bringing out the trash! Only kidding.

Transition / Perineal.

Foetal head on perineum (crowning), then emerging. Great deal of pressure and stretching, some women describe a burning and stinging sensation in the perineum. If you feel this, some caregivers recommend that you stop pushing for a few minutes to allow the tissue to stretch and open gradually, breath slowly and deeply. I found a little counter pressure helpful.

Positions for Pushing

The most common position for second stage in most hospitals is semi-sitting (a distinct improvement over the lithotomy position with feet up in stirrups that was common in the 1950's and 60's.) However, research and anthropological evidence have found advantages to other, more upright positions. An ideal position would: open the pelvic outlet as widely as possible, provide a smooth path for the baby to descend through the birth canal, use the advantages of gravity to help the baby move down, and give the mother a sense of being safe and in control of the process.

Try out a position for a few contractions. If it works, stay with it. If not, switch to a new position in between contractions. If you're like me, you'll probably go through every known position until you're comfortable!

> Changing positions is good not only for the mother's comfort, but also to change the shape of the birth canal to help the baby make the required movements prior to birth, and to ensure on-going oxygen supply to the foetus.

Spontaneous Bearing Down.

When you feel the urge to push, you will feel your uterus contracting, and can try to work with it. When you feel a contraction coming on, tuck your chin, curl your shoulder forward, and open your legs wider. When you feels the urge to push, gently bear down and push. Stop pushing when the urge passes.

Directed Pushing.

For a mom without the urge to push, a caregiver will observe when she's having a contraction (by watching the monitor if in hospital, or by resting a hand on mom's belly), and will coach her on when to push. When a contraction begins, mom takes a deep breath in and releases it, then takes in another deep breath, tucks chin and bears down for six seconds. She gently pushes downward with abdominal muscles, while visualizing the baby moving down and out. (Some women exhale while pushing, others may hold their breath for five to seven seconds. It may help to grunt or vocalize while exhaling.) Then she relaxes and takes a few breaths, then bears down again. Generally, do about 3 pushes per contraction, following the urge to push when possible.

Laboring Down / Delayed Pushing.

Some caregivers recommend that mothers with no urge to push, and particularly mothers with an epidural in place, just rest and relax. They recommend waiting to actively push until baby is crowning at the perineum; this may be an hour or more after you reach 10 cm dilation. Labouring down will lead to a longer second stage than a more active, directed pushing, but it's not as exhausting, and some studies have shown that it leads to fewer instrumental deliveries. Some caregivers are not familiar with this method. If you and your baby are doing well, and tolerating labour well, you may ask if this is an option for you. This is similar to how I breathed out my third baby, but I had a midwife familiar with alternative birthing,

How to Avoid Pushing, if necessary.

Some women may feel an urge to push at only 8 to 9 cm. Research indicates that involuntary pushing is not harmful at this stage if 1) the cervix is soft and retracting, 2) the foetal station is 0 to +1 or more, 3) the baby is transverse or anterior. However, you don't want to be pushing actively at this point, so your caregiver may tell you not to push. Also, during crowning, while you're pushing the baby out, the doctor may occasionally ask you to stop pushing. It is very difficult to convince your uterus to stop pushing at this point!

However, you can do all you can to not actively push.

If your caregiver has told you that you need to pause in pushing, this breathing technique may help reduce the urge to push. Lift your chin, lean back, and arch your back a little. Pant, blowing lightly. Visualize a feather, and blow just enough to keep the feather bouncing up and down in the air above your lips.

How hard to push.

Enough to push the pain away and maintain the feeling of being open but not so much that you produce additional pain. It's better to think of yourself "opening" and "helping the baby move down" and "easing the baby out" than to think of "pushing."

Making Noise.

Many women have the instinctive need to vocalize during pushing: grunts and low-pitched groans. These are a natural part of the effort of pushing, and should be welcomed and encouraged by partners.

If you feel like practicing for the Second Stage. First of all, empty your bladder. Get into a semi-sitting position, either propped up by a few pillows, or in your partner's arms. Place your hands beneath the lower curve of your abdomen; partner can also place his hands there by reaching around you. Take in a deep breath and hold it for six seconds (holding your breath for longer than this can be dangerous for your baby, as it reduces the oxygen content of the blood.) Drop your chin forward onto your chest, and allow the bulge beneath your hands to press downward and forward, pushing your hands out and forward. You will feel your perineum move too, bulging very gently outward, and then the tissues of the vagina spreading out. Then exhale and relax.

This can also be practiced while sitting on the toilet, using a chamomile steam bath, as this is where you are familiar with releasing pelvic floor muscles. Or it can be practiced in other birthing positions. Inhale, put chin on chest, and curl body forward; bear down *gently* as if having a bowel movement, pressing from the inside steadily out, slowly and gently; then exhale and relax. The goal of this practice is to release the muscles and feel what the relaxation of those muscles feel like. Do not practice hard pushing!!

After practice, do some Kegel exercises to tone your pelvic floor muscles.

Practice a few times a week. These are those muscles your birth teacher will tell you to use after the birth.

Third Stage: Delivering the Placenta

The third stage begins when the baby is born. It is when the placenta separates from the wall of the uterus, and is delivered through the vaginal canal.

You will still be having contractions at this time, but they are much less intense than before and you may not notice them. For some women, especially if it's not the first time giving birth, they're still strong enough that it helps to use labour breathing techniques to cope with the discomfort of these contractions. Some women are so enraptured with the baby that they barely notice the cramping.

Your caregiver may ask you to push a few times to deliver the placenta. Again, this pushing is less intense than the delivery of the baby. Or sometimes your midwife will just push down on your belly and plop.....!

Third stage usually lasts ten to thirty minutes. If it lasts longer than this, you may be given Pitocin to increase contractions to encourage the delivery of the placenta, and help the uterus to begin involution (shrinking back down to the non-pregnant size.)

During third stage is also the time when your caregiver will clean your genital area, examine your perineum, and will stitch up your perineum if you've torn or had an episiotomy. A local anaesthetic is used if you haven't had an epidural.

In this period after birth, most of the parents' attention centres on the baby, and not so much on the final stage of labour. In the first hour after birth, you will want to begin breastfeeding. Breastfeeding with help get your tummy back to prepregnancy shape, and it creates a bond with your baby. For me it was the most natural reaction in the world to put my baby to my breast. I used to really enjoy breastfeeding, it was so special, and that little tiny face looking up at me, with little tiny clenched fists!

If you have problems breastfeeding because of infections, like mastitis, my wonderful midwife made the following compress for me. I got a breast infection after every birth, and it helped immensely.

Get a towel or wide bandage and spread it with a whole tub of quark, that cream cheese stuff. Now wrap this around your breasts, both of them, and leave it for as long as possible. Massaging your breasts from underarm or outwards towards the nipple. This helps empty the breast of all extra milk.

How will labor be induced?

Sometimes Mother Nature needs a little prodding. A first time mother often goes over her due date, but when she goes over more than two weeks, labour will normally be induced or a section will be performed. If you are wondering how they will induce, here are a few examples along with a short explanation of each.

Stripping the membranes

Stripping the membranes is where a doctor or midwife separates your bag of water from the cervix, it is not intended to break your water, however it may. It may also cause infection, and may be painful for some.

Pitocin

This is an artificial version of the body's hormone oxytocin. It is given by IV and is used to cause contractions. The amount of Pitocin used will depend on how your body accepts it. Generally, the amount is increased every 15-30 minutes until a good contraction pattern is achieved. Sometimes this is done in combination with breaking the bag of water

Prostaglandin Gels/Suppositories

These are used more frequently when the cervix is not favourable, meaning that it is dilated less than 3 centimetres, hard, posterior, not effaced, or barely effaced, or any combination of the above. This can be used alone, or more frequently will be done 12 or more hours prior to the use of Pitocin. Frequently it will be given more than once over the course of an evening/night. A suppository or tampon like substance will be placed in or near your cervix during a vaginal exam.

Misoprostal

This is a pill that can either be ingested orally or placed near the cervix. It is used more often when the cervix is not very favourable.

If like me you don't savour the thought of a hospital induction, you could try the following cocktail. This is a tried and trusted old time European method to induce labour. I don't know if the origins are in witchcraft, but I know it works. On my third child, in fear of ending up in hospital for birth I used this with success, and know of many many more women who have also used this. But be warned! Only ever use this if you go over your due date! It will not work if you have not yet gone over your due date as your body is not yet ready and shouldn't be pushed into going into labour if it is not ready. And it should be done before going to bed.

Rizinuscocktail:

First make a cup of black coffee, and leave it on your bedside table.

Wrap a hot water bottle in a towel and place in the bed

Now mix the following.

4 tablespoons of castor oil

4 tablespoons of orange or apricot juice

4 tablespoons of cognac.

You must drink this cocktail in one go while lying in bed. Directly afterwards, drink the black coffee as fast as you can without burning yourself and then go to sleep. You will awake at about two in the morning with contractions. If done correctly, you will experience absolutely NO loose bowel movements!

Another method to naturally induce labour would be to have intercourse with your partner. Sperm is known to induce labour in a woman with a ripe cervix.

Aromatherapy: ginger, vervain, cinnamon and clove can stimulate labour. Try either a bath with 10 drops of one of the oils.

A belly massage with 5 drops oil to 150ml carrier oil.

Herbal teas: a stick of cinnamon, a small ginger root, 10 cloves, tablespoon vervain. In a litre of water and sweetened with honey. Drink the full litre during a 24 hour period, lukewarm!

Homeopathy: globules which can help induce labour; Caulophyllum, Cimcifuga, Kalium carbonicum, Nux vomica, Pulsatilla, Sepia. Ask your midwife or homeopath for advice.

Bibliography

Further reading

'Homeopathy for Mother and Baby' Miranda Castro, Macmillan

'Homeopathic Medicines for Pregnancy and Childbirth' Richard Moskowitz MD, North Atlantic Books

'Homoeopathy for Babies and Children, a parents' guide' Beth MacEoin, Hodder and Stoughton Headway

Gypsy Sorcery and Fortune Telling by Charles Godfrey Leland (1891)

S

T

V

Other Books by Jennifer Meier

Diagon 2

The House of Elizabeth Gass

ISBN 978-1-4461-2632-5

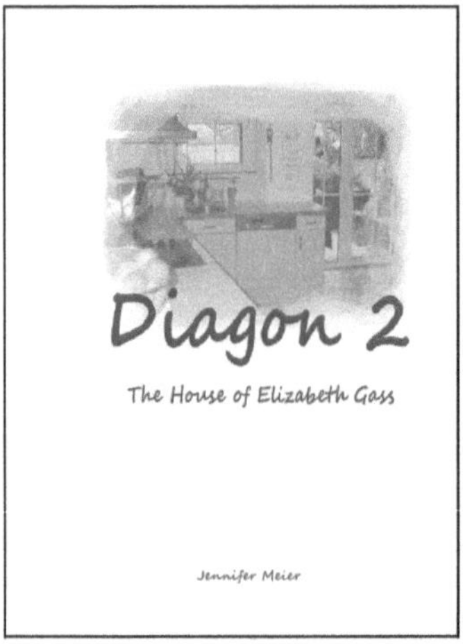

After moving to a new country, Nicki has finally found happiness, but that peace seems destined to be drowned under the rage of a long dead man. Growing up amongst the superstitious Irish, Nicki is used to tales of Ghosts and otherworld creatures, but nothing prepared her for what was waiting on her within the walls of her newly bought home. She had long ago fallen into the arms of traditional Witchcraft, and only her belief in the world of magic and Ghosts keeps her sane while she tries to come to terms with her childhood fear and solve the riddle that has been placed upon her shoulders.

Ollie Learns English
ISBN 978-1-4461-2522-9

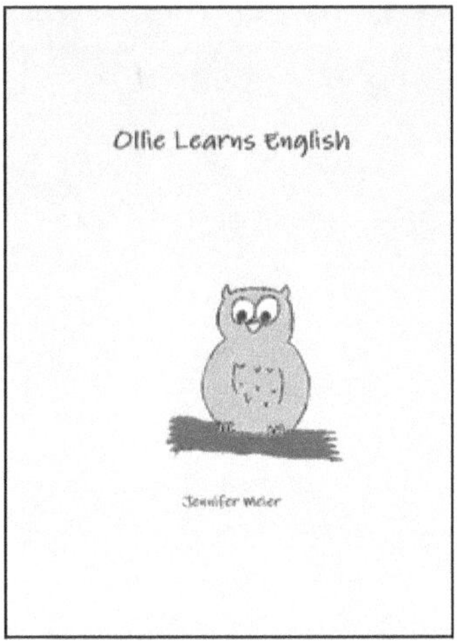

Learning English as a foreign language for native German speaking children. Lots to colour and make throughout the year while having as much fun as possible.

www.ingramcontent.com/pod-product-compliance
Lightning Source LLC
Chambersburg PA
CBHW061255280526
45784CB00002B/774
9781446126011